Ernst Schering Research Foundation Workshop
Supplement 9
Testicular Tangrams

Springer
Berlin
Heidelberg
New York
Barcelona
Hong Kong
London
Milan
Paris
Tokyo

Ernst Schering Research Foundation Workshop
Supplement 9

Testicular Tangrams

12th European Workshop on Molecular and Cellular Endocrinology of the Testis

F.F.G. Rommerts, K.J. Teerds
Editors

With 29 Figures

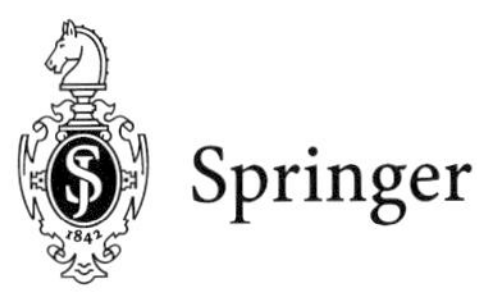

Springer

Series Editors: G. Stock and M. Lessl

ISSN 1431-7133
ISBN 3-540-43255-8   Springer-Verlag Berlin Heidelberg New York

Die Deutsche Bibliothek - CIP-Einheitsaufnahme
Testicular tangrams / 12th European Testis Workshop 2002. Ernst Schering Research Foundation.
Focko F. G. Rommerts and Katerine J. Teerds. - Berlin ; Heidelberg ; New York ; Barcelona ; Hongkong ; London ; Milan ; Paris ; Tokyo : Springer, 2002
(Ernst Schering Research Foundation Workshop : Supplement ; 9)
 ISBN 3-540-43255-8

Springer-Verlag Berlin Heidelberg New York
a member of BertelsmannSpringer Science+Business Media GmbH

http://www.springer.de

Typesetting: Data conversion by Springer-Verlag
Printing: Druckhaus Beltz, Hemsbach.
Binding: J. Schäffer GmbH & Co. KG, Grünstadt
SPIN: 10865460   21/3130/AG–5 4 3 2 1 0 – Printed on acid-free paper

Preface

During the past two decades research on the testis has created a vast number of publications. New techniques, such as cell and gene cloning, germ cell manipulation and transplantation, as well as gene expression, have surpassed the classical approaches that involved studies on receptor activation and endocrine, paracrine and autocrine regulatory mechanisms. Due to the expansion of this field of research it has become increasingly difficult to integrate the large number of observations and relate them to the physiology and pathophysiology of the testis. More emphasis must, therefore, be put on the integration of isolated findings and the construction of the total picture. In order to stimulate this specific mental activity we have named this book ***Testicular Tangram***. We hope that the chapters in this book will be used as pieces of the testicular puzzle and that the reader enjoys composing new shapes.

The chapters of this book are representative of the plenary lectures presented at the 12th European Workshop on Molecular and Cellular Endocrinology of the Testis held in Doorwerth The Netherlands, from April 6 - 10, 2002. Publication of this book has been made possible by the generous support of the Ernst Schering Research Foundation. We would also like to thank the distinguished scientists, who have provided us with their excellent manuscripts well before the start of the Workshop. We acknowledge the help of Dr. U.-F. Habenicht, Dr. M. Lessl, Ms W. McHugh and the members of the local organizing committee, as listed below, in the preparation of this book.

Focko Rommerts and Katja Teerds

Local organizing committee

Ben Colenbrander
Federica M. F. van Dissel-Emiliani
Focko F.G. Rommerts
Dirk G. de Rooij
Katja J. Teerds
Axel P.N. Themmen

Contents

List of Editors and Contributors

Editors

F.F.G. Rommerts
Department of Internal Medicine, Erasmus University Rotterdam, Rotterdam,
The Netherlands (e-mail: rommerts@endov.fgg.eur.nl)

K. Teerds
Department of Biochemistry and Cell Biology, Faculty of Veterinary Medicine, Utrecht University, P.O. Box 80176, 3508 TD Utrecht, The Netherlands
(e-mail: k.j.teerds@vet.uu.nl)

Contributors

J.C. Achermann
Division of Endocrinology, Metabolism and Molecular Medicine,
Northwestern University, Medical School, Chicago, IL 60611-3072, USA
(e-mail: j-achermann@northwestern.edu)

T. Ashley
Department of Genetics, Yale University School of Medicine,
333 Cedar Street, New Haven, CT 06510, USA
(e-mail: terry.ashley@yale.edu)

R. Bars
Aventis CropScience, 355 Rue Dostoievski, BP 153, 06903 Sophia-Antipolis,
France

M. Benahmed
Institut National de la Santé et de la Recherche Médical, U. 407,
Faculté de Medicine Lyon-Sud, BP12, 69921 Oullins Cedex, France
(e-mail: benahmed@lsgrisnl.univ-lyonl.fr)

L. Benbrahim-Tallaa
Institut National de la Santé et de la Recherche Médical, U. 407,
Faculté de Medicine Lyon-Sud, BP 12, 69921 Oullins Cedex, France

A. Bozec
Institut National de la Santé et de la Recherche Médical, U. 407,
Faculté de Medicine Lyon-Sud, BP 12, 69921 Oullins Cedex, France

L.B. Creemers
Department of Cell Biology, UMCU, and Department of Endocrinology,
Faculty of Biology, H. R. Kruytgebouw, Padulaan 8, 3584 CH Utrecht,
The Netherlands (e-mail: L.B.Creemers@lab.azu.nl)

F. Chuzel
Aventis CropScience, 355 Rue Dostoievski, BP 153, 06903 Sophia-Antipolis,
France

F. Fanelli
Dipartimento di Chimica, Università di Modena e Reggio Emilia,
via Campi 183, 41100 Modena, Italy (e-mail: fanelli@unimo.it)

L.P. Freedman
Cell Biology Program, Memorial Sloan-Kettering Cancer Center,
1275 York Avenue, New York, NY 10021, USA
(e-mail: l-freedman@ski.mskcc.org)

A. Florin
Institut National de la Santé et de la Recherche Médical, U.407,
Faculté de Medicine Lyon-Sud, BP 12, 69921 Oullins Cedex, France

M.D. Griswold
School of Molecular Biosciences, Center for Reproductive Biology,
Washington State University, Pullman, Washington, USA
(e-mail: griswold@mail.wsu.edu)

I. Goddard
Institut National de la Santé et de la Recherche Médical, U.407,
Faculté de Medicine Lyon-Sud, BP 12, 69921 Oullins Cedex, France

I. Huhtaniemi
Department of Physiology, University of Turku, Kiinamyllynkatu 10,
20520 Turku, Finland (e-mail: ilpo.huhtaniemi@utu.fi)

R. Ivell
Institute for Hormone and Fertility Research, University of Hamburg,
Grandweg 64, 22529 Hamburg, Germany (e-mail: ivell@ihf.de)

F. Izadyar
Department Cell Biology, UMCU, and Department of Endocrinology,
Faculty of Biology, H.R. Kruytgebouw, Padulaan 8, 3584 CH Utrecht,
The Netherlands (e-mail: fizadyar@lab.azu.nl)

J.L. Jameson
Department of Medicine, NUMS/NMH Galter Pavillon, Suite 3-150,
251 E.Huron St. Chicago, IL 60611-2908, USA
(e-mail: ljameson@northwestern.edu)

C. Mauduit
Institut National de la Santé et de la Recherche Médical, U. 407,
Faculté de Medicine Lyon-Sud, BP 12, 69921 Oullins Cedex, France

D. McLean
School of Molecular Biosciences, Center for Reproductive Biology,
Washington State University, Pullmann, Washington, USA
(e-mail: dmclean@wsunix.wsu.edu)

J.J. Meeks
Division of Endocrinology, Metabolism and Molecular Medicine,
Northwestern University, Medical School, Chicago, IL 60611-3072, USA
(e-mail: j-meeks@northwestern.edu)

Y. Nishimune
Department of Science for Laboratory Animal Experimentation, Research In-
stitute for Microbial Diseases, Osaka University, 3-1 Yamadaoka, Suita City,
Osaka 565-0871, Japan (e-mail: nishimun@biken.osaka-u.ac.jp)

M. Nozaki
Department of Science for Laboratory Animal Experimentation, Research Institute for Microbial Diseases, Osaka University, 3-1 Yamadaoka, Suita City, Osaka 565-0871, Japan (e-mail: mnozaki@biken.osaka-u.ac.jp)

A. Omezzine
Institut National de la Santé et de la Recherche Médical, U407, Faculté de Medicine Lyon-Sud, BP 12, 69921 Oullins Cedex, France

K. den Ouden
Department of Cell Biology, UMCU, and Department of Endocrinology, Faculty of Biology, H.R. Kruytgebouw, Padulaan 8, 3584 CH Utrecht, The Netherlands (e-mail: k.denouden@lab.azu.nl)

G. Oziski
Division of Endocrinology, Metabolism and Molecular Medicine, Northwestern University, Medical School, Tarry 15, 303 E. Chicago Avenue, Chicago, IL 60611-3072, USA (e-mail: gokhan@northwestern.edu)

M. Poutanen
Department of Physiology, University of Turku, Kiinamyllynkatu 10, 20520 Turku, Finland

D.G. de Rooij
Department Cell Biology, UMCU, and Department of Endocrinology, Faculty of Biology, H.R. Kruytgebouw, Padulaan 8, 3584 CH Utrecht, The Netherlands (e-mail: d.g.derooij@med.uu.nl)

A.-N. Spiess
Insitute for Hormone and Fertility Research, University of Hamburg, Grandweg 64, 22529 Hamburg, Germany (e-mail: spiess@ihf.de)

E. Tabone
Institut National de la Santé et de la Recherche Médical, U407, Faculté de Medicine Lyon-Sud, BP 12, 69921 Oullins Cedex, France

H. Tanaka
Department of Science for Laboratory Animal Experimentation, Research Institute for Microbial Diseases, Osaka University, 3-1 Yamadaoka, Suita City, Osaka 565-0871, Japan (e-mail: tanaka@biken.osaka.u.ac.jp)

D.J. Wolgemuth
Department of Genetics and Development, Columbia University College of
Physicians and Surgeons, 630 West 168th Street, Lab BB, Black Building
1613, New York, NY 10032, USA (e-mail: djw3@columbia.edu)

K. Yomogida
Department of Science for Laboratory Animal Experimentation, Research In-
stitute for Microbial Diseases, Osaka University, 3-1 Yamadaoka, Suita City,
Osaka 565-0871, Japan (e-mail: yomo@biken.osaka-u.ac.jp)

F.-P. Zhang
Institute of Biomedicine and Physiology, University of Helsinki,
Haarmanikatu 8, 00014 Helsinki, Finland (e-mail: fuping.zhang@helsinki.fi)

1 Multiple Guardians of the Epithelial Stage IV Meiotic Checkpoint

T. Ashley

Cell cycle checkpoints and checkpoint proteins monitor the condition of the DNA and chromosomes as they proceed through their appointed rounds (Hartwell and Weinert 1989). "Monitoring" includes detecting irregularities, such as replication arrest, DNA lesions or chromosomes unattached to the spindle. Once an abnormality has been detected, the damage surveillance network of cell cycle proteins halts cell cycle progression until the error is rectified, or shunts the cell into an apoptotic pathway. The location and function of somatic cell cycle checkpoints have been the subject of extensive investigations and are well defined (Murray and Hunt 1993; Weinert and Lydall 1993; Elledge 1996; Hoekstra 1997; Weinert 1997; Stillman 1999). They include a G1 checkpoint, an intra-S checkpoint, a G2 checkpoint and an M checkpoint. The G1 checkpoint assures that there is no unrepaired damage to the DNA as the cell begins to replicate and the checkpoint proteins set in motion replication of genes required for DNA synthesis. Similarly the G2 checkpoint ensures that there is no unrepaired damage as the cell prepares to divide. The intra S checkpoint monitors both progression of DNA replication and any DNA damage such as double strand breaks (DSBs). In the event of a break, the intra S checkpoint halts replication until repair is completed. In contrast to the other checkpoints, the M checkpoint is a spindle checkpoint that assures all the chromosomes are attached to the spindle and oriented to opposite poles. If an error in a somatic cell cannot be remedied, eliminating the cell prevents the perpetuation of the error. The same is true in meiotic cells. However, if the error is due to a mutation in a critical gene required for meiosis and all the affected spermatocytes undergo apoptosis, the consequence is male sterility (see (Ashley 2000) for a recent review).

Much less is known about meiotic checkpoints: their location within meiosis, their function, and their protein composition has remained an enigma. The fact that mammalian meiosis is an extremely protracted event that occurs over a two-week period in mice (Oakberg 1957) provides a high degree of temporal resolution and recent studies on meiotic progression, or more accurately lack of progression, in mice in which critical genes have been disrupted have pinpointed the time of their arrest during spermatogenesis. The discovery of this checkpoint in male mice and the identification of some of the protein components associated with it are the subject of this paper. The finding that these meiotic prophase proteins are the same as those involved in the mitotic intra S phase checkpoint not only allows us to infer their role in meiosis, but also provides new insights on early meiotic prophase events.

1.1 Mutations That Trigger a Meiotic Checkpoint

Targeted disruption, or "knock-out" of specific genes has become a powerful tool for study of gene function. *Atm*, the gene mutated in the human autosomal recessive disorder, ataxia telangiectasia, is a cell cycle protein involved in the detection of double strand breaks (DSBs) (Meyn 1995; Shiloh 1995). ATM appears to be involved in the G1, the intra S and the G2 checkpoints (Hoekstra 1997; Westphal 1997; Shiloh 2001). Mice homozygous recessive (knocked-out) for *Atm* are male sterile with the arrest occurring during meiotic prophase (Barlow, Hirotsune et al. 1996; Xu, Ashley et al. 1996). Homologous chromosomes initiate synapsis, but the synapsed bivalents fragment (Xu, Ashley et al. 1996). The onset of fragmentation does not coincide with the commencement of synapsis, but is slightly delayed such that there is usually extensive synapsis within the spermatocyte (Xu, Ashley et al. 1996). Nonetheless, in most nuclei many chromosomes, or parts of chromosomes remain asynapsed. A report of a very early prophase – i.e. leptotene disruption in *Atm-/-* spermatocytes (Barlow, Liyanage et al. 1997), was apparently due to the authors' inability to distinguish between the formation of axial elements in early meiotic prophase and apoptotic nuclei in which similar pieces of axes are all that remain.) According to the classic definition of meiotic prophase stages, the presence of asynapsed autosomal segments in these cells would dictate that these cells be considered to be in zygonema. (Completion of homologous synapsis of the entire autosomal complement is considered the transition from zygonema to pachynema). However, analysis of testis sections indicates that these spermatocytes proceeded to Epithelial Stage IV before arresting (D.G. de Rooij, personal communication). Spermatocytes in normal mouse testis at Stage IV have reached mid-pachynema (Oakberg 1956; Oakberg 1957; de Rooij and Grootegoed 1998). Thus histological analysis of testis sections provides a more accurate estimate of the actual age and physiological stage of the spermatocytes than does cytological examination.

The tenuous link between meiotic arrest at Epithelial Stage IV and synaptic failure was strengthened considerably when two asynaptic mutants were found to arrest at this stage (de Vries, Baart et al. 1999). DMC1 is a recA/Rad51 meiotic-specific homolog required for establishment of interhomolog interactions required for meiotic synapsis and recombination (Bishop, Park et al. 1992; Pittman, Cobb et al. 1998; Yoshida, Kondoh et al. 1998). MSH 5 is a meiotic specific mismatch repair protein (Hollingsworth, Ponte et al. 1995), and is also required for establishment of interhomolog interactions and meiotic synapsis in mammals (de Vries, Baart et al. 1999; Edelmann, Cohen et al. 1999). Spermatocytes in *Dmc1-/-* mice are largely asynaptic (Pittman, Cobb et al. 1998; Yoshida, Kondoh et al. 1998), as are those from *Msh5-/-* (de Vries, Baart et al. 1999; Edelmann, Cohen et al. 1999).

1.2 Proteins That Localize to Sites Along Asynapsed Axes

Immunohistochemical studies of normal mice have resulted in localization of several proteins to asynapsed autosomal axes during zygonema. These include ATR (Keegan, Holtzman et al. 1996), Rad51 (Plug, Xu et al. 1996), BRCA1 (Scully, Chen et al. 1997), and BRCA2 (Chen, Silver et al. 1998). ATR is a ortholog of ATM (Cimprich, Shin et al. 1996; Keegan, Holtzman et al. 1996) and has recently been shown to be an intra S phase checkpoint protein (Brown and Baltimore 2000; Tibbetts, Cortez et al. 2000). Rad51 is a mammalian homologue of recA, a bacterial protein that binds to single-stranded DNA and plays a key role in recombination (Kowalczykowski 1991; Radding 1991). Although Rad51 appears to play a similar role in eukaryotes (Robu, Inman et al. 2001), it has recently been suggested that it may also bind to ssDNA at stalled replication forks (Aguilera 2001). BRCA1 (Scully, Chen et al. 1997) and BRCA2 (Mizuta, LaSalle et al. 1997; Chen, Silver et al. 1998; Patel, Yu et al. 1998; Chen, Silver et al. 1999) were originally assumed to be involved in recombination, based largely on their association with RAD51. However, BRCA1 is phosphorylated by ATR when replication is blocked by hydroxyurea (Tibbetts, Cortez et al. 2000), and now appears to be a component of an intra-S checkpoint. To summarize, several proteins that have been shown to localize to asynapsed axes have been implicated in a mitotic intra S checkpoint that detects the presence of unreplicated DNA and halts cell cycle progression until the damage is repaired. These include ATR and BRCA1. In addition it has been suggested that RAD51 may bind to ssDNA at delayed replication forks. BRCA1 may not be able to directly interact with RAD51, but can only do so through BRCA2 (Chen, Chen et al. 1998), suggesting that BRCA2 must be either a direct, or indirect component of the checkpoint. In support of a critical role of all of these genes in DNA replication (rather than occasional repair) in somatic cells, targeted disruption of any of these genes leads to early embryonic lethality: Rad51 (Lim and Hasty 1996; Tsuzuki, Fujii et al. 1996; Sharan, Morimatsu et al. 1997), BRCA1 (Gowen, Johnson et al. 1996; Liu, Flesken-Nikitin et al. 1996; Shen, Weaver et al. 1998), BRCA2 (Ludwig, Chapman et al. 1997; Sharan, Morimatsu et al. 1997) and ATR (Brown and Baltimore 2000).

1.3 Connections Between the Stage IV Checkpoint and the Proteins at Sites Along Asynapsed Axes

The arrest of the *Atm-/-* spermatocytes originally presented a curious dilemma. If a checkpoint gene is mutated, the mutation is expected to result in an abrogation of the checkpoint. Yet the *Atm-/-* spermatocytes arrested rather than bypassing this meiotic checkpoint. Since the putative checkpoint proteins on the asynapsed axes (BRCA1 and BRCA2 and ATR) lead to embryonic lethality when disrupted, their effect on the meiotic checkpoint cannot be easily assessed. Yet the fact that all of these proteins are now known to be involved in the mitotic intra S checkpoint offers an interesting explanation. In somatic tissues this intra S checkpoint is a "dual" checkpoint that monitors both progression of replication and DNA damage. ATM has also been shown to be a component of this checkpoint in mitotic cells (Meyn 1995; Lavin and Khanna 1999; Shiloh 2001) as evidenced by the fact that cells from individuals with ataxia telangiectasia do not halt replication when gamma irradiation produces DSBs (Painter 1981; Painter 1993). However, BRCA1 and ATR are also components of this checkpoint (Tibbetts, Cortez et al. 2000). Their continued presence along the asynapsed axes in *Atm-/-* spermatocytes raises the interesting possibility that a replication-associated process may remain incomplete in these cells. Consistent with this interpretation of the Stage IV checkpoint being of a dual nature that that monitors both damage and replication with detection of either type of error resulting in arrest, immunohistochemical analysis of cytological preparations of spermatocytes from *Atm-/-* mice revealed ATR remained at sites along the asynapsed autosomal segments even as the synapsed portions underwent wide-spread fragmentation (Plug, Peters et al. 1997). In addition, RPA remains at sites along the synapsed axes and fragmentation occurred at the RPA sites (Plug, Peters et al. 1997).

Extensive analysis of *Dmc1-/-* mice has revealed that ATR, RAD51, BRCA1 and BRCA2 all remain at many sites along the asynapsed axes in these spermatocytes (Walpita, de Magio, and Ashley, unpublished observations).

1.4 Additional Checkpoint Proteins Whose Time of Appearance and Disappearance Are Consistent with Involvement in the Stage IV Checkpoint

The components of the MRE11, RAD50, and NBS1 (mammals) or Xrs2 (*S. cerevisiae*) complex were originally identified as "repair proteins" (Johzuka and Ogawa 1995). Consistent with this repair role, MRE11 has exonuclease activity and is involved in the 3′ to 5′resection of DSBs (Nairz and Klein 1997; Paull and Gellert 1998; Trujillo, Yuan et al. 1998; Tsubouchi and Ogawa 1998). Rare individuals that are homozygous recessive for a mutation in the human *Mre11* gene have DNA repair defects similar to individuals with ataxia-telangiectasia (Stewart, Maser et al. 1999). Mutations in Rad50 and Xrs1 in yeast (Ivanov, Korolev et al. 1992; Raymond and Kleckner 1993; Bressan, Baxter et al. 1999; Chamankahah and Xiao 1999), or RAD50 and NBS1 in mammals (Trujillo, Yuan et al. 1998; Ito, Tauchi et al. 1999; Paull and Gellert 1999) are also repair defective. Mutations in NBS1 are responsible for another rare autosomal recessive disorder – Nijmegen Breakage Syndrome (Varon, Vissinga et al. 1998; Digweed, Reis et al. 1999). Similar to individuals with the *Mre11* mutation, these individuals share DNA repair defects similar to individuals with ataxia telangiectasia. It has recently become apparent that these genetic disorders share more than defective repair with ataxia telangiectasia. The Mre11/Rad50/Xrs2 complex in yeast (D'Amours and Jackson 2001; Grenon, Gilbert et al. 2001) and the MRE11/RAD50/NBS1 complex in humans (Sullivan, Veksler et al. 1997; Carney, Maser et al. 1998) are also components of the intra S phase checkpoint. In fact, when DSBs are induced, NSB1 is a phosphorylation target of ATM (Wu, Ranganathan et al. 2000).

In yeast the Rad50/Mre11/Xrs2 complex has not only been shown to be essential for meiosis (Ivanov, Korolev et al. 1992; Johzuka and Ogawa 1995; Nairz and Klein 1997; Ohta, Nicolas et al. 1998; Tsubouchi and Ogawa 1998), but mutations in these genes in yeast are asynaptic (Alani, Padmore et al. 1990; Loidl, Klein et al. 1994; Weiner and Kleckner 1994). In mammals, deletion of the RAD50 (Xiao and Weaver 1997; Luo, Yao et al. 1999), MRE11 (Xiao and Weaver 1997), and NBS1 (Zhu, Petersen et al. 2001) all result in embryonic lethality. Information on the effects of mutation of specific sites within these genes is not yet available. However, antibodies against RAD50 and MRE11 have been localized in mouse spermatocytes (Goedecke, Eijpe et al. 1999; Eijpe, Offenberg et al. 2000). Unlike RAD51 and BRCA1, BRCA2, RPA and the other proteins discussed above, antibodies to the members of the MRE11 complex do not produce foci in meiotic prophase (Goedecke, Eijpe et al. 1999; Eijpe, Offenberg et al. 2000 and Plug and Ashley, unpublished observations). However, in testis sections, the antibodies produce a general chromatin reaction from around premeiotic S phase until around Epithelial Stage 4 which corresponds to around midpachynema of meiotic prophase (Goedecke, Eijpe et al. 1999; Eijpe, Offenberg et al. 2000). Thus these mitotic intra S checkpoint genes are not only present during meiotic prophase, but their disappearance corresponds to the Stage IV checkpoint.

1.5 What Is the Relationship Between the Somatic Intra-S Phase Checkpoint and the Meiotic Epithelial Stage IV Checkpoint?

There are two obvious similarities between the mitotic intra-S checkpoint and the Stage IV meiotic checkpoint: the dual nature of the checkpoint (replication and damage detection) and the checkpoint proteins they share. In somatic cells it is easy to understand why the intra-S checkpoint includes detection of both types of errors (incomplete replication and damage). In fact it is becoming increasingly evident that in addition to the long recognized hazards of extrinsic damage, DSBs at "stalled forks" are an intrinsic problem associated with normal eukaryotic DNA replication (Courcelle and Hanawalt 2001; Kuzminov 2001). Thus detection and repair of DSBs is a critical component of DNA replication.

In meiotic cells, programmed DSBs during early meiotic prophase have long been recognized as an early step in meiotic synapsis and recombination (see (Roeder 1990; Kleckner and Weiner 1993; Roeder 1997) for review). Although there is a tendency to automatically consider meiotic prophase "post-replicative", one model of meiotic synapsis predicts that a small amount of DNA remains unreplicated until early meiotic prophase (see (Plug, Xu et al. 1996; Ashley and Plug 1998; Ashley 2000) for review). The delayed replication model is based on the work Hotta and Stern who found that a small fraction of the genome of lily (0.1–0.3%) was not replicated during premeiotic S phase, but delayed in replication until homologous chromosomes synapse (Hotta, Ito et al. 1966; Hotta and Stern 1971). If replication of these sequences is chemically blocked, homologues do not synapse and the chromosomes eventually fragment (Ito, Hotta et al. 1967). Although the delayed replication model has long been out of favor, recent evidence that synapsis involves a different repair pathway than does recombination (Allers and Lichten 2001; Hunter and Kleckner 2001) has resulted in a revival of interest in this model. An intra-S meiotic checkpoint could be predicted as an essential component of this delayed replication model of meiotic synapsis.

As discussed above, in somatic cells ATR appears to monitor progression of replication. In these cells if DNA synthesis is arrested ATR phosphorylates BRCA1 (Tibbetts, Cortez et al. 2000) although BRCA1 is also phosphorylated by ATM in the presence of DSBs (Cortez, Wang et al. 1999; Gatei, Scott et al. 2000). In this respect it is instructive to note that ATR, BRCA1, BRCA2 and RAD51 all localize at sites along *asynapsed* axes, before the *Atm-/-* data suggest that DSBs occur. As mentioned above, RAD51 has recently been found to bind to ssDNA including replication forks at sites between unreplicated and already replicated DNA (Aguilera 2001). The RAD51 foci on asynapsed axes have been postulated to represent ssDNA, not of individual regions of resected ssDNA, but multiple ssDNA regions corresponding to unreplicated replication clusters (Plug, Xu et al. 1996). Furthermore, RAD51 (Plug, Xu et al. 1996), BRCA1, BRCA2 and ATR [(Scully, Chen et al.

1997; Chen, Silver et al. 1998) and Plug and Ashley, unpublished observations] are often found at corresponding sites on the asynapsed axes, a localization consistent with delayed replication of the same sequences on the two homologues. The colocalization of BRCA1 with ATR, but not ATM suggests that the meiotic role of BRCA1 is more similar to its somatic role at arrested replication forks, than in the DSB pathway. The most parsimonious explanation for the colocalization of these proteins is that they are all associated with sequences that have been delayed in their replication until homologous chromosomes begin to synapse.

Unlike the situation in yeast, the mammalian genome is full of repetitive sequences and the chance of illegitimate recombination is high. Therefore it would seem that the meiotic system would have evolved to maximize the probability of repair from a homologous chromosome A check for homology in meiotic nuclei that precedes the formation of double strand breaks would provide this opportunity. The fragmentation of synapsed, but not asynapsed chromosomes, in *Atm-/-* spermatocytes (Xu, Ashley et al. 1996) is certainly consistent with this assumption. ATM has recently been shown to phosphorylate NBS1 following DSB damage in an intra S checkpoint in somatic cells (Lim, Kim et al. 2000). MRE11 has also been found to prevent accumulation of DSBs during replication in somatic cells. How does the NBS1/MRE11/RAD50 complex fit into the intra S checkpoint cascade? Recent evidence suggests that this complex is involved in a repair process known as break induced replication (Kuzminov 2001; Rattray, McGill et al. 2001; Signon, Malkova et al. 2001). This repair pathway is emerging as the primary pathway used by somatic cells to restart DNA synthesis when replication forks collapse (see Kuzminov 2001 for review).

1.6 If Homologous Chromosomes Synapse During Zygonema, Why Is the Synaptic Checkpoint Temporally Located in Mid-Pachynema?

We have seen that there is one set of proteins located on asynapsed axes: RAD51, BRCA1, BRCA2 and ATR. As homologues synapse, another set of proteins that have been implicated in the replication process appears at corresponding sites on the synapsed axes: RPA and ATM (Plug, Peters et al. 1997), and BLM (Walpita, Plug et al. 1999). RPA is a ssDNA binding protein that is required for both replication and repair (Coverley and Laskey 1994; Umezu, Sugawara et al. 1998; Iftode, Daniely et al. 1999; Walter and Newport 2000). In mouse spermatocytes it is present at sites along synapsed chromosomes as soon as they synapse. Although the number of total sites begins to decrease shortly after synapse, some sites remain until around mid-pachynema. It has been suggested that RPA is involved in the processing (i.e. replication) of the RAD51-associated sequences (Plug, Peters et al. 1997; Plug, Peters et al. 1998). RAD51 and RPA briefly colocalize on newly synapsed axes (Plug, Peters et al. 1998). Although the evidence is circumstantial, the disappearance of RPA would seem to coincide with the completion of replication. It is unlikely to be a coincidence that RPA disappearance appears to roughly coincide with the Stage IV checkpoint.

As mentioned above, the disappearance of MRE11 and RAD50 in testis sections also occurs during meiosis around Stage IV (Goedecke, Eijpe et al. 1999; Eijpe, Offenberg et al. 2000).

1.7 Is Reciprocal Recombination (Crossover) Monitored by the Epithelial Stage IV Checkpoint?

Since reciprocal recombination is almost certainly initiated by DSBs (Szostak, Orr-Weaver et al. 1983; Cao, Alani et al. 1990; Kleckner, Padmore et al. 1991), this step is likely to be monitored by the Stage IV checkpoint. Only one unique protein component of the reciprocal recombination repair pathway has been identified: MLH1 (Baker, Plug et al. 1996; Hunter and Borts 1997). MLH1 foci colocalize with a subset of RPA in early meiotic prophase, but persist long after the disappearance of RPA (Plug, Peters et al. 1998). In some stains of mice MLH1 remain on spermatocyte synaptonemal complexes until near the end of pachynema (Baker, Plug et al. 1996); in others they remain into diplonema, where they localize to chiasmata sites (Webb and Ashley, unpublished observations), suggesting that the monitoring of completion of crossover is not Stage IV checkpoint control. Consistent with this assumption, spermatocytes from *Mlh1-/-* are achiasmatic and arrest at

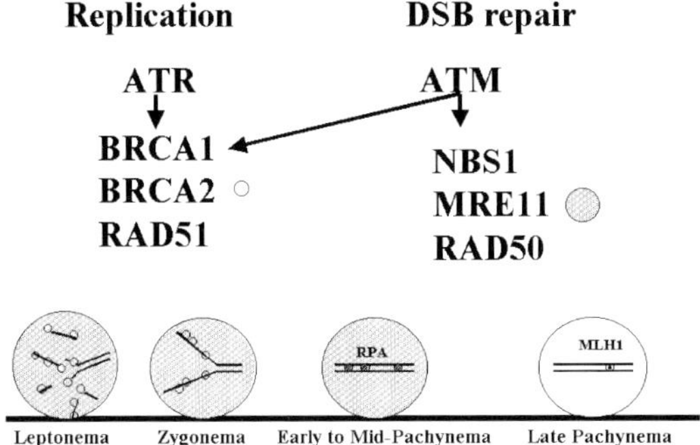

Fig. 1. The *upper portion* of the diagram shows the known interactions of the proteins in somatic cells. The *lower portion* shows their distribution during meiotic prophase

metaphase I (Baker, Plug et al. 1996). Apparently the univalents are "caught" by a spindle checkpoint at this stage. If the disappearance of MLH1 is any indication, the completion of crossover occurs long after Stage IV (Fig. 1).

1.8 Summary

In summary, the meiotic Stage IV checkpoint appears to be associated with completion of molecular events associated with synapsis. The continuing presence of one set of intra S phase checkpoint proteins (ATR, BRCA1 and BRCA2) on asynapsed axes and the disappearance of another set of intra S phase checkpoint proteins (Mre11/RAD50/NBS1) around Stage IV of meiotic prophase, the most likely "molecular event" is DNA replication. This interpretation is consistent with the emerging evidence that the homologous recombination pathway is not the mechanism of the meiotic check for homology and synapsis.

References

Aguilera, A. (2001). "Double-strand break repair: are Rad51/RecA–DNA joints barriers to DNA replication?" *Trends Genet* **17**: 318–321.

Alani, E., R. Padmore, et al. (1990). "Analysis of wild-type and *rad50* mutants of yeast suggests an intimate relationship between meiotic chromosome synapsis and recombination." *Cell* **61**: 419–436.

Allers, T. and M. Lichten (2001). "Differential timing and control of noncrossover and crossover recombination during meiosis." *Cell* **106**: 47–57.

Ashley, T. (2000). An integration of old and new perspectives of mammalian meiotic sterility. *Results and Problems in Cell Differentiation: The Genetic Basis of Male Infertility*. K. McEcelreay. Berlin, Heidelberg, Springer-Verlag. **28**: 131–173.

Ashley, T. and A. W. Plug (1998). Caught in the act: deducing meiotic function from protein immunolocalization. *Current Topics in Dev Biol*. M. A. Handel, Academic Press. **37**: 201–239.

Baker, S. M., A. W. Plug, et al. (1996). "Involvement of mouse *Mlh1* in DNA mismatch repair and meiotic crossing over." *Nat Genet* **13**: 336–342.

Barlow, C., S. Hirotsune, et al. (1996). "Atm-deficient mice: a paradigm of ataxia telangiectasia." *Cell* **86**: 159–171.

Barlow, C., M. Liyanage, et al. (1997). "Partial rescue of the prophase I defect of Atm-deficient mice by p53 and p21 null alleles." *Nat Genet* **17**: 462–466.

Bishop, D. K., D. Park, et al. (1992). "*DMC1*: a meiotic specific yeast homolog of *E. coli* recA required for recombination, synaptonemal complex formation and cell cycle progression." *Cell* **69**: 439–456.

Bressan, D. A., B. K. Baxter, et al. (1999). "The Mre11-Rad50-Xrs2 protein complex facilitates homologous recombination-based double-strand break repair in *Saccharomyces cerevisiae*." *Mol Cell Biol* **19**: 7681–7687.

Brown, E. J. and D. Baltimore (2000). "ATR disruption leads to chromosomal fragmentation and early embryonic lethality." *Genes Dev* **15**: 397–402.

Cao, L., E. Alani, et al. (1990). "A pathway for generation and processing of double-strand breaks during meiotic recombination in *S. cerevisiae*." *Cell* **61**: 1089–1101.

Carney, J. P., R. S. Maser, et al. (1998). "The hMre11/hRad50 protein complex and Nijmegen breakage syndrome: linkage of double-strand break repair to the cellular DNA damage response." *Cell* **93**: 477–486.

Chamankahah, M. and W. Xiao (1999). "Formation of the yeast Mre11-Rad50-Xrs2 complex is correlated with DNA repair and telomere maintenance." *Nucl Acid Res* **27**: 2072–2079.

Chen, J., D. P. Silver, et al. (1998). "Stable interactions between the products of the *BRCA1* and *BRCA2* tumor suppressor genes in mitotic and meiotic cells." *Molec Cell* **2**: 317–328.

Chen, J. J., D. P. Silver, et al. (1999). "BRCA1, BRCA2, and Rad51 operate in a common damage response pathway." *Cancer Res* **57**: 1752–1756.

Chen, P., C. F. Chen, et al. (1998). "The BRC repeats in BRCA2 are critical for RAD51 binding and resistance to methyl methanesulfonate treatment." *Proc Natl Acad Sci USA* **95**: 5287–5292.

Cimprich, K. A., T. B. Shin, et al. (1996). "cDNA cloning and gene mapping of a candidate human cell cycle checkpoint protein." *Proc Natl Acad Sci USA* **93**: 2850–2855.

Cortez, D., Y. Wang, et al. (1999). "Requirement of ATM-dependent phosphorylation of BRCA1 in the DNA damage response to double-strand breaks." *Science* **286**: 1162–1166.

Courcelle, J. and P. C. Hanawalt (2001). "Participation of recombination proteins in rescue of arrested replication forks in UV-irradiated *Escherichia coli* need not involve recombination." *Proc Natl Acad Sci USA* **98**: 8196–8202.

Coverley, D. and R. A. Laskey (1994). "Regulation of eukaryotic DNA replication." *Annu Rev Biochem* **63**: 745–776.

D'Amours, D. and S. P. Jackson (2001). "The yeast Xrs2 complex functions in S phase checkpoint regulation." *Genes Dev* **15**: 2238–2249.

de Rooij, D. G. and J. A. Grootegoed (1998). "Spermatogonial stem cells." *Curr Opin Cell Biol* **10**: 694–701.

de Vries, S. S., E. B. Baart, et al. (1999). "Mouse MutS-like protein MSH5 is required for proper chromosome synapsis in male and female meiosis." *Genes Dev* **13**: 523–531.

Digweed, M., A. Reis, et al. (1999). "Nijmegen breakage syndrome: consequences of defective DNA double-strand break repair." *Bioessays* **21**: 649–656.

Edelmann, W., P. E. Cohen, et al. (1999). "Mammalian MutS homolgue 5 is required for chromosome pairing in meiosis." *Nat Genet* **21**: 123–127.

Eijpe, M., H. Offenberg, et al. (2000). "Localization of Rad50 and MRE11 in spermatocyte nuclei of mouse and rat." *Chromosoma* **109**: 123–132.

Elledge, S. J. (1996). "Cell cycle checkpoints: preventing an identity crisis." *Science* **274**: 1664–1672.

Gatei, M., S. P. Scott, et al. (2000). "Role for ATM in DNA damage-induced phosphorylation of BRCA1." *Cancer Res* **60**: 3299–3304.

Goedecke, W., M. Eijpe, et al. (1999). "MRE11 and Ku70 interact in somatic cells, but are differentially expressed in early meiosis." *Nat Genet* **23**: 194–198.

Gowen, L. C., B. L. Johnson, et al. (1996). "*Brca1* deficiency results in early embryonic lethality characterized by neuroepithelial abnormalities." *Nat Genet* **12**: 191–194.

Grenon, M., C. Gilbert, et al. (2001). "Checkpoint activation in response to double-strand breaks requires the Mre11/Rad50/Xrs2 complex." *Nat Cell Biol* **3**: 844–847.

Hartwell, L. H. and T. A. Weinert (1989). "Checkpoints: controls that ensure the order of cell cycle events." *Science* **249**: 629–634.

Hoekstra, M. F. (1997). "Responses to DNA damage and regulation of cell cycle checkpoints by the ATM protein kinase family." *Curr Op in Gen Dev* **7**: 170–175.

Hollingsworth, N. M., L. Ponte, et al. (1995). "MSH5, a novel MutS homolog, facilitates meiotic reciprocal recombination between homologs in *Saccharomyces cerevisiae* but not mismatch repair." *Genes Dev* **9**: 1728–1739.

Hotta, Y., M. Ito, et al. (1966). "Synthesis of DNA during meiosis." *Proc Natl Acad Sci USA* **56**: 1184–1191.

Hotta, Y. and H. Stern (1971). "Analysis of DNA synthesis during meiotic prophase in *Lilium*." *J Mol Biol* **55**: 337–355.

Hunter, N. and R. H. Borts (1997). "Mlh1 is unique among mismatch repair proteins in its ability to promote crossing-over during meiosis." *Genes Dev* **11**: 1573–1582.

Hunter, N. and N. Kleckner (2001). *Cell* **106**: 59–70.

Iftode, C., Y. Daniely, et al. (1999). "Replication protein A (RPA): the eukaryotic SSB." *Crit Rev Biochem Mol Biol* **34**: 141–180.

Ito, A., H. Tauchi, et al. (1999). "Expression of full-length NBS1 protein restores normal radiation responses in cells from Nijmegen breakage syndrome patients." *Biochem Biophys Res Commun* **265**: 716–721.

Ito, M., Y. Hotta, et al. (1967). "Studies of meiosis in vitro. II. Effect of inhibiting DNA synthesis during meiotic prophase on chromosome structure and behavior." *Dev Biol* **16**: 54–77.

Ivanov, E. L., V. G. Korolev, et al. (1992). "XRS2, a DNA repair gene of *Saccharomyces cerevisiae*, is needed for meiotic recombination." *Genetics* **132**: 651–664.

Johzuka, K. and H. Ogawa (1995). "Interaction of mre11 and Rad50: two proteins required for DNA repair and meiosis-specific double-strand break formation in *Saccharomyces cerevisiae*." *Genetics* **139**: 1521–1532.

Keegan, K. S., D. A. Holtzman, et al. (1996). "The ATR and ATM protein kinases associate with different sites along meiotically pairing chromosomes." *Genes Dev* **10**: 2423–2437.

Kleckner, N., R. Padmore, et al. (1991). "Meiotic chromosome metabolism: one view." *Cold Spring Harbor Symp Quant Biol* **56**: 729–743.

Kleckner, N. and B. M. Weiner (1993). "Potential advantages of unstable interactions for pairing of chromosomes in mitotic, somatic and premeiotic cells." *Cold Spring Harbor Symp Quant Biol* **58**: 553–565.

Kowalczykowski, S. C. (1991). "Biochemical and biological function of Escheria coli RecA protein: behavior of mutant RecA proteins." *Biochimie* **73**: 289–304.

Kuzminov, A. (2001). "DNA replication meets genetic exchange: chromosomal damage and its repair by homologous recombination." *Proc Natl Acad USA* **98**: 8461–8468.

Lavin, M. F. and K. K. Khanna (1999). "ATM: the protein encoded by the gene mutated in the radiosensitive syndrome ataxia-telangiectasia." *Int J Radiat Biol* **75**: 1201–1214.

Lim, D.-S. and P. Hasty (1996). "A mutation in mouse *rad51* results in an early embryonic lethal that is suppressed by a *p53* mutation." *Mol Cell Biol* **16**: 7133–7143.

Lim, D. S., S. T. Kim, et al. (2000). "ATM phosphorylates p95/Nbs1 in an S-phase checkpoint pathway." *Nature* **404**: 613–617.

Liu, C.-Y., A. Flesken-Nikitin, et al. (1996). "Inactivation of the mouse *Brca1* gene leads to failure in the morphogenesis of the egg cylinder in early postimplantation development." *Genes Dev* **10**: 1835–1843.

Loidl, J., F. Klein, et al. (1994). "Homologous pairing is reduced but not abolished in asynaptic mutants of yeast." *J Cell Biol* **125**: 1191–1200.

Ludwig, T., D. L. Chapman, et al. (1997). "Targeted mutations of breast cancer susceptibility gene homologs in mice: lethal phenotypes of *Brca1, Brca2, Brca1/Brca2, Brca1/p53, and Brca2/p53* nullizygous embryos." *Genes Dev* **11**: 1226–1241.

Luo, G. B., M. S. Yao, et al. (1999). "Disruption of mRad50 causes embryonic stem cell lethality, abnormal embryonic development, and sensitivity to ionizing radiation." *Proc Natl Acad Sci USA* **96**: 7376–7381.

Meyn, M. S. (1995). "Ataxia-telangiectasia and cellular responses to DNA damage." *Cancer Res* **55**: 5991–6001.

Mizuta, R., J. M. LaSalle, et al. (1997). "RAB22 and RAB163/mouse BRCA2: proteins that specifically interact with the RAD51 protein." *Proc Natl Acad Sci USA* **94**: 6927–6932.

Murray, A. W. and T. Hunt (1993). *The Cell Cycle: An Introduction.* New York, Oxford University Press.

Nairz, K. and F. Klein (1997). "mre11S– a yeast mutation that blocks double-strand-break processing and permits nonhomologous synapsis in meiosis." *Genes Dev* **11**: 2272–2290.

Oakberg, E. F. (1956). " A description of spermatogenesis in the mouse and its use in analysis of the cycle of the seminiferous epithelium." *Am J Anat* **99**: 507–516.

Oakberg, E. F. (1957). "Duration of spermatogenesis in the mouse." *Nature* **180**: 1137–1138.

Ohta, K., A. Nicolas, et al. (1998). "Mutations in the MRE11, RAD50, XRS2, and MRE2 genes alter chromatin configuration at meiotic DNA double-stranded break sites in premeiotic and meiotic cells." *Proc Natl Acad Sci USA* **95**: 646–651.

Painter, R. B. (1981). "Radioresistant DNA synthesis: an intrinsic feature of ataxia telangiectasia." *Mutat Res* **84**: 183–190.

Painter, R. B. (1993). Radiobiology of ataxia-telangiectasia. *Ataxia-telangiectasia*. R. A. Gatti and R. B. Painter. Heidelberg, Springer-Verlag: 257–268.

Patel, K. J., V. P. Yu, et al. (1998). "Involvement of *Brca2* in DNA repair." *Mol Cell* **1**: 347–357.

Paull, T. T. and M. Gellert (1998). "The 3′ to 5′ exonuclease activity of Mre11 facilitates repair of DNA double-strand breaks." *Mol Cell* **1**: 969–979.

Paull, T. T. and M. Gellert (1999). "Nbs1 potentiates ATP-driven DNA unwinding and endonuclease cleavage by the Mre11/Rad50 complex." *Genes Dev* **13**: 1276–1288.

Pittman, D. L., J. Cobb, et al. (1998). "Meiotic prophase arrest with failure of chromosome synapsis in mice deficient for *Dmc1*, a germline-specific RecA homolog." *Mol Cell* **1**: 697–705.

Plug, A. W., A. H. F. M. Peters, et al. (1997). "ATM and RPA in meiotic chromosome synapsis and recombination." *Nat Genet* **17**: 457–461.

Plug, A. W., A. H. F. M. Peters, et al. (1998). "Changes in protein composition of meiotic nodules during mammalian meiosis." *J Cell Sci* **111**: 413–423.

Plug, A. W., J. Xu, et al. (1996). "Presynaptic association of RAD51 protein with selected sites in meiotic chromatin." *Proc Natl Acad Sci USA* **93**: 5920–5924.

Radding, C. M. (1991). "Helical interactions in homologous pairing and strand exchange driven by RecA protein." *J Biol Chem* **266**: 5355–5358.

Rattray, A. J., C. B. McGill, et al. (2001). "Fidelity of mitotic double-strand break repair in *Saccharomyces cerevisiae*: a role for *SAE2/COM1*." *Genetics* **158**: 109–122.

Raymond, W. E. and N. Kleckner (1993). "RAD50 protein of *S. cerevisiae* exhibits ATP-dependent DNA binding." *Nucleic Acids Res* **21**: 3851–3856.

Robu, M. E., R. B. Inman, et al. (2001). "RecA protein promotes the regression of stalled forks *in vitro*." *Proc Natl Acad Sci USA* **98**: 8211–8218.

Roeder, G. S. (1990). "Chromosome synapsis and genetic recombination." *Trends Genet* **6**: 385–389.

Roeder, G. S. (1997). "Meiotic chromosomes: it takes two to tango." *Genes Dev* **11**: 2600–2621.

Scully, R., J. Chen, et al. (1997). "Association of BRCA1 with RAD51 in mitotic and meiotic cells." *Cell* **88**: 265–275.

Sharan, S. K., M. Morimatsu, et al. (1997). "Embryonic lethality and radiation hypersensitivity mediated by *Rad51* in mice lacking *Brca2*." *Nature* **368**: 804–810.

Shen, S. X., Z. Weaver, et al. (1998). " A targeted disruption of the murine *Brca1* gene causes gamma-irradiation hypersensitivity and genetic instability." *Oncogene* **17**: 3115–3124.

Shiloh, Y. (1995). "Ataxia-telangiectasia: Closer to unraveling the mystery." *Eur J Hum Genet* **3**: 116–138.

Shiloh, Y. (2001). "ATM and ATR: network in cellular responses to DNA damage." *Curr Opin Genet Dev* **11**: 71–77.

Signon, L., A. Malkova, et al. (2001). "Genetic requirements for *RAD51*- and *Rad54*-independent break-induced replication repair of a chromosomal double-strand break." *Mol Cell Biol* **21**: 2048–2056.

Stewart, G. S., R. S. Maser, et al. (1999). "The DNA double-strand break repair gene hMre11 is mutated in individuals with an ataxia-telangiectasia-like disorder." *Cell* **99**: 577–587.

Stillman, B. (1999). "Cell cycle control of DNA replication." *Science* **274**: 1659–1664.

Sullivan, K. E., E. Veksler, et al. (1997). "Cell cycle checkpoints and DNA repair in Nijmegen breakage syndrome." *Clin Immunol Immunopathol* **82**: 43–48.

Szostak, J. W., T. L. Orr-Weaver, et al. (1983). "The double-strand-break repair model for recombination." *Cell* **33**: 25–35.

Tibbetts, R. S., D. Cortez, et al. (2000). "Functional interactions between BRCA1 and the checkpoint kinase ATR during genotoxic stress." *Genes Dev* **14**: 2989–3002.

Trujillo, K. M., S. S. F. Yuan, et al. (1998). "Nuclease activities in a complex of human recombination and DNA repair factors RAD50, MRE11, and p95." *J Biol Chem* **273**: 21447–21450.

Tsubouchi, H. and H. Ogawa (1998). "A novel *mre11* mutation that impairs processing of double-strand breaks of DNA during both mitosis and meiosis." *Mol Cell Biol* **18**: 260–268.

Tsuzuki, T., Y. Fujii, et al. (1996). "Targeted disruption of the Rad51 gene leads to lethality in embryonic mice." *Proc Natl Acad Sci USA* **93**: 6236–6240.

Umezu, K., N. Sugawara, et al. (1998). "Genetic analysis of yeast RPAI reveals its multiple functions in DNA metabolism." *Genetics* **148**: 989–1005.

Varon, R., C. Vissinga, et al. (1998). "Nibrin, a novel DNA double-strand break repair protein, is mutated in Nijmegen breakage syndrome." *Cell* **93**: 467–476.

Walpita, D., A. W. Plug, et al. (1999). "Bloom's syndrome protein (BLM) colocalizes with RPA in meiotic prophase nuclei of mammalian spermatocytes." *Proc Natl Acad Sci USA* **96**: 5622–5627.

Walter, J. and J. Newport (2000). "Initiation of eukaryotic DNA replication: origin unwinding and sequential chromatin association of Cdc45, RPA, and DNA polymerase α." *Mol Cell* **5**: 617–627.

Weiner, B. M. and N. Kleckner (1994). "Chromosome pairing via multiple interstitial interactions before and during meiosis in yeast." *Cell* **77**: 977–991.

Weinert, T. (1997). "A DNA damage checkpoint meets the cell cycle engine." *Science* **277**: 1450–1451.

Weinert, T. and D. Lydall (1993). "Cell cycle checkpoints, genetic instability and cancer." *Cancer Biol* **4**: 129–140.

Westphal, C. H. (1997). "Atm displays its many talents." *Current Biol* **7**: 789–792.

Wu, X., V. Ranganathan, et al. (2000). "ATM phosphorylation of Nijmegen breakage syndrome protein is required in a DNA damage response." *Nature* **405**: 477–482.

Xiao, Y. H. and D. T. Weaver (1997). "Conditional gene targeted deletion by Cre recombinase demonstrates the requirement for the double strand break repair gene Mre11 protein in murine embryonic stem cells." *Nucl Acid Res* **25**: 2985–2991.

Xu, Y., T. Ashley, et al. (1996). "Targeted disruption of ATM leads to growth retardation, chromosomal fragmentation during meiosis, immune defects, and thymic lymphoma." *Genes Dev* **10**: 2411–2422.

Yoshida, K., G. Kondoh, et al. (1998). "The mouse RecA-like gene DMC1 is required for homologous chromosome synapsis during meiosis." *Mol Cell* **1**: 707–718.

Zhu, J., S. Petersen, et al. (2001). "Targeted disruption of the Nijmegen breakage syndrome gene NSB1 leads to early embryonic lethality in mice." *Curr Biol* **11**: 105–109.

2 Role of Sertoli Cells in Hypospermatogenesis Induced by Antiandrogens

M. Benahmed, F. Chuzel, R. Bars, A. Omezzine, C. Mauduit,
L. Benbrahim-Tallaa, I. Goddard, A. Bozec, A. Florin, E. Tabone

2.1 Introduction

Environmental chemicals which mimic or antagonize the actions of steroid hormones have the potential to disrupt endocrine function and could potentially pose a threat to human health [1–3]. Different studies have documented the ability of these chemicals to interfere with male gonadal formation and function in experimental models [4, 5]. As steroid hormones play a critical role in the early development of the genital tract [6], it has been hypothesized that some synthetic chemicals in the environment could affect adult male reproductive organs by stimulating or inhibiting receptor mediated developmental events following an in utero exposure [5]. Several reports in the literature have indicated that in utero exposure to exogenous anti-androgenic compounds can induce a wide range of abnormalities of the reproductive system, including small testes, cryptorchidism and hypospadia [5–8]. These compounds have been reported to interact with the androgen receptor [7, 8]. For example, the drug flutamide and its active metabolite hydroxyflutamide are non-steroidal synthetic chemicals able to inhibit the action of androgens at the receptor level [9]. In utero exposure to flutamide has been shown to induce major alterations in the accessory sex glands and in testis development in male rat offspring [5–8]. Exposure to this antiandrogen resulted in a decrease in the gonad weight with marked testicular morphological alterations including a reduction in average diameter of the seminiferous tubules associated with moderate to severe hypospermatogenesis with an interruption of germ cell maturation [8]. The cellular and molecular mechanisms underlying the arrest of the spermatogenetic process resulting in the loss of the mature germ cells remain to be investigated.

In this brief review, we present some data issued mainly from our laboratory indicating that such a hypospermatogenesis is related to an apoptotic process occurring in germ cells and which is probably initiated in Sertoli cells, the target cells of androgens in the seminiferous tubules.

2.2 Germ Cell Depletion in Adult Rat Testis Exposed In Utero to Flutamide Is Related to an Apoptotic Cell Death Process

In the adult rat testis exposed in utero to flutamide (0.4, 2, 10 mg/kg/day), a reduction in average diameter of the seminiferous tubules with moderate to severe hypospermatogenesis depending on the dose of the antiandrogen was observed. At 10 mg/kg/day, an arrest of germ cell maturation was clearly observed. This spermatogenetic process appears to be related to a cell death process as shown by the TUNEL approach. Indeed, while in control untreated animals, very few if any TUNEL-positive cells were observed in the testes, TUNEL-positive cells were clearly identified in adult rat testis exposed in utero to flutamide. These positive cells were mainly located to meiotic and post-meiotic germ cells. No TUNEL-positive cells were detected in somatic

(Leydig and Sertoli) cells nor in spermatogonia at the different doses of flutamide administered in utero. The number of apoptotic germ cells increased in a flutamide dose dependent manner. The number of Sertoli cells was not affected [10)].

The number of cells in an organ is determined by the rates of cell migration, cell division and cell death [11]. The phenomenon of cell death has been discovered independently several times over the past 150 years (for references, see [12]). Cell death in multicellular organisms is subject to genetic control and abnormalities in cell death regulation can cause diseases such as cancer, autoimmunity and possibly degenerative disorders. Four major functional groups of molecules involved in triggering and affecting apoptosis process have been identified. These are caspases, the adaptator proteins which control the activation of initiator caspases, members of the tumor necrosis factor (TNF) receptor (TNFR) super family, and members of the Bcl-2 family of proteins. The family of cysteine proteases called caspases (at least 14 caspases have been identified in mammals) play a central role in the execution of programmed cell death by cleaving a wide variety of substrates leading to the characteristic morphological changes associated with apoptosis. Caspases could be divided into two types – those with large prodomains that function upstream as initiators of death cascade (e.g. caspases-2, -9, -8) and those with a small prodomain that act downstream as effectors (e.g. caspases 10, 3, 6 and 7).

In order to characterize the germ cell death apoptotic process occurring in rat testis exposed in utero to flutamide, we have initially focussed our approach on caspases and more specifically on three types of caspases : caspase-3, -6 and –8 [10].

In the adult rat testis, caspase-3 immunostaining was specifically detected in germ cells but not in somatic cells. Caspase-3 immunostaining is predominantly observed in pachytene spermatocytes. This observation is compatible with that of Kim et al [13]. The intensity of caspase-3 immunostaining increased along with the different doses of flutamide administered in utero, including 0.4, 2 and 10 mg/kg/day. Similarly, in the adult rat testis exposed in utero to flutamide (0.4, 2, and 10 mg/kg/day), caspase-3 mRNA levels increased in a flutamide dose dependent manner. The maximal increase in caspase-3 mRNA levels was observed at 2 mg/kg/day. A parallel flutamide dose dependent increase in procaspase-3 protein levels was observed. As for caspase-3, caspase-6 immunostaining was detected in germ cells but not in somatic cells. Caspase-6 immunostaining was predominantly observed in pachytene spermatocytes. In the adult rat testis exposed in utero to flutamide, the intensity of caspase-6 immunostaining increased along with the different doses of flutamide. Caspase-6 mRNA levels were also enhanced in a flutamide dose dependent manner. The increase in caspase-6 mRNA was accompanied by a parallel and flutamide dose dependent increase in procaspase-6 protein levels. As for caspase-3 and –6, caspase-8 immunostaining was predominantly observed in pachytene spermatocytes . However, caspase-8 immunostaining was found to be not affected in adult rats exposed in utero to flutamide. Consistently, no changes occurred in caspase 8 mRNA and protein levels [10].

Together, these data indicate that exposure to flutamide occurring in utero induced a permanent increase in the expression of caspase-3 and -6 (but not of caspase-8) in the adult rat testis. These observations support therefore a relationship between expression of caspases-3, -6 but not caspase-8 and androgen action.

Sertoli cells are the direct target cells to testosterone action since they are the unique cells that express androgen receptor (AR) in the in the seminiferous tubules. These observations would suggest that the permanent apoptotic process associated with the increased caspase 3 and 6 mRNA and protein levels occurs in the context of germ cell- Sertoli cell interactions under the androgen control. Therefore, it is possible that following in utero exposure to flutamide, alterations leading to germ cell apoptosis occur primarily in Sertoli cells. Although the nature of Sertoli cell intermediates involved in germ cell apoptosis are at present time unknown, growth factors and cytokines could be interesting candidates. Indeed, these factors are known to be antiapoptotic factors and some of these factors are produced in Sertoli cells under hormonal control and their receptors are expressed in germ cells [for review, (14)]. However, the possibility also exists that other factors and other mechanisms might be at play. In general, the factors originating from Sertoli cells and controlling germ cell survival remain to be identified.

The mechanisms, the molecules as well as the signalling systems that trigger apoptosis in germ cells following alterations of Sertoli cell activity resulting from antiandrogen action remain to be investigated. Here, we suggest at least two possibilities where Sertoli cell activity could be affected: (i) alteration of the detoxification systems (decrease of glutathione S-transferase α) which protect germ cells and (ii) alteration of the energy metabolism through the decrease in the production and transport of lactate, an energy substrate produced by Sertoli cells and required for germ cell development.

2.3 Glutathione S-Transferase α Expression in Sertoli Cells Is Reduced in Adult Rat Testis Exposed In Utero to Flutamide

The glutathione S-transferases (GSTs) (EC 2.5.1.18) belong to a supergene family of phase II detoxification enzymes that catalyze the nucleophilic addition of glutathione to the electrophilic centers of a wide variety of xenobiotics [15–17]. They also serve as transport proteins for a broad range of lipophilic compounds, such as steroid hormones [18]. Cytosolic, microsomal and nuclear forms of GSTs have been identified in different tissues. The cytosolic GSTs exist as homodimers or heterodimers and are separated into several classes (alpha, mu, pi, sigma and theta) based on the degree of homology of their subunits [15–20].

In the testis, the protective functions of GSTs are especially crucial for germ cells, in which electrophilic compounds and reactive oxygen intermediates could have profound effects on sperm formation and motility, and are potentially hazardous to the integrity of germ cell DNA [21, 22]. For example, in addition to its role as phase II detoxification enzymes involved in the conjugation of electrophilic xenobiotics such as carcinogens and mutagens to the endogenous nucleophile GSH, GSTα contributes also, particularly in the testis, to a major portion of the selenium-independent glutathione peroxidase (GPx) activity toward phosphatidylcholine hydroperoxide [15–20]. GSTα may be therefore necessary to protect this tissue from reactive oxygen species-induced damage. The importance of GSTs in the protection against oxidative stress in testes is underscored by recent studies showing that when GST activity is inhibited, accumulation of products of lipid peroxidation is augmented, resulting in germ cell apoptosis [23]. More recently, these observations were further strengthened by data demonstrating that overexpression of GSTA2–2 (a member of GSTα class) in K562 cells attenuates the cytotoxic effect of H_2O_2 and other oxidants and protects against H_2O_2-induced apoptosis by blocking caspase 3 activation [24]. Therefore, an alteration in the detoxifying process related to a permanent decrease in the expression of GSTα in the seminiferous tubules may provide one of the bases of explanation for the hypospermatogenesis (due to an increased apoptosis process?) observed in adult rats exposed in utero to the antiandrogen.

A permanent alteration of the expression of glutathione S-transferase α (GSTα), was evidenced in the rat testis exposed in utero to the antiandrogen. Testicular GSTα was shown to be immunoexpressed exclusively in somatic Leydig and Sertoli cells. Following an in utero exposure to flutamide, GSTα immunostaining decreased in Sertoli cells but not in Leydig cells. Such a decrease in GSTα immunoexpression in Sertoli cells occurred at the GSTα mRNA levels. This decrease in GSTα mRNA levels was correlated to a parallel and comparable decrease in GSTα protein levels in Sertoli cells. The reduction in GSTα expression in the adult rat Sertoli cells following an in utero exposure to flutamide was not related to a decrease in Sertoli cell number nor to testosterone and/or AR deficiency. Indeed, circulating testosterone and LH levels in the adult rats and AR immunoexpression in Sertoli cells were not affected in adult animals exposed in utero to flutamide [25]. Together, these observations indicate that the inhibition of testosterone activity by androgen receptor blockage in the fetal life renders the activity of Sertoli cells partly or totally unresponsive to androgen action. More specifically, the action of testosterone on GSTα expression in rat testis exposed in utero to the antiandrogen appears to be compromised downstream the AR. Assuming the key role of the GSTs in the detoxifying processes in different tissues including the testis, the decrease in GSTα mRNA and protein in the seminiferous tubules may provide one of the bases of explanation for the hypospermatogenesis observed in the adult rats exposed in utero to flutamide.

2.4 Lactate Production and Transport Are Decreased in Adult Rat Testis Exposed In Utero to Flutamide

We have also investigated the hypothesis that in the adult rat testis exposed in utero to flutamide, germ cell death could be related to defects in energy metabolism and particularly to defects of the production and transport of lactate. Lactate is a preferential energy substrate produced by Sertoli cells and transported to germ cells by monocarboxylate transporters (MCT). A significant decrease (60%) in lactate production was observed in cultured Sertoli cells from rat testes exposed in utero to flutamide. Such a decrease is concurrent to a decrease in LDH A mRNA levels and LDHA activity. The decrease in LDHA mRNA levels (to 64 ± 9% of the control) was observed with a low dose (2 mg/kg/day) of flutamide tested. The decrease in LDH A mRNA levels was observed in both the whole testis and in isolated Sertoli cells, suggesting that such a decrease in LDHA expression occurred also in the cells producing lactate. Lactate is transported from Sertoli cells to germ cells via MCT1 and MCT2. We (immuno)localized MCT1 to all the different germ cell types and MCT2 exclusively to elongated spermatids. In the adult testis exposed in utero to flutamide, MCT1 and MCT2 mRNA levels were significantly reduced indicating that lactate transport to germ cells was also altered. For example, in the adult rat exposed in utero to 10 mg/kg/day of flutamide, MCT1 and MCT2 mRNA levels were reduced to 53±8% and 52±9%, respectively. Alterations of the immunoexpression of MCT1 and MCT2 were observed in adult rat testis exposed in utero to a higher dose (10 mg/kg/day) of flutamide (Goddard et al). Together, these data support (i) the existence of a relationship between the antiandrogen activity and the energy metabolism in the testis, (ii) the concept of an androgen-dependent programming, occurring early in fetal life in relation to the expression of some of the key genes involved in the production and transport of lactate in the seminiferous tubules and (iii) that the reduction of both the production of lactate by Sertoli cells as well as the transport of this energy metabolite to germ cells may explain, at least partly, the germ cell apoptotic cell death observed in adult rat testis exposed in utero to flutamide.

Together, the data presented here indicate that the hypospermatogenesis observed in the adult rat testis exposed in utero to the antiandrogen flutamide might be related to an increased permanent apoptotic cell death process which affects pachytene spermatocytes and post meiotic germ cells. Such a process is probably initiated in Sertoli cells. The activity but not the number of Sertoli cells is affected. The mechanisms involved in the alterations of Sertoli cell activity remain to be investigated. We suggest, however, at least two potential alterations in Sertoli cell activity which might be linked to the apoptotic germ cell death: (i) an alteration of the detoxification processes such as a decrease in Sertoli cell GSTα expression and (ii) changes in the energy metabolism through a decrease in lactate production and transport.

References

1. Cheek AO, McLachlan JA (1998) Environmental hormones and the male reproductive system. J Androl 19:5–10.
2. Ashby J, Houthoff E, Kennedy SJ, Stevens J, Bars R, Jekat FW, Campbell P, Van Miller J, Carpanini FM, Randall GL (1997) The challenge posed by endocrine-disrupting chemicals. Environ Health Perspect 105:164–169.
3. Crisp TM, Cleeg ED, Cooper RL, Anderson DG, Baetcke KP, Hoffman JL, Morrow MS, Rodier DJ, Schaeffer JE, Touart LW, Zeeman MG, Patel YM, Wood WP (1997) Special report on environmental endocrine disruption: an effect assessement and analysis.
4. Colborn T, vom Saal FS, Soto AM (1993) Developmental effects of endocrine-disrutping chemicals in wildlife and humans. Env Health Perspectives 101:378–384
5. Sharpe RM, Fisher JS, Saunders PT, Lajdig G, Millar MR, Parte P, Kerr JB, Turner KJ (1998) Estrogen effects on development and function of the testis. Germ cell developpement, division, disruption and death, Massachussets.
6. Kelce WR, Wilson EM(1998) Developmental effects and mechanisms of environmental antiandrogens. Germ cell development, division, disruption and death., Massachussets.
7. Jost A, Vigier B, Prepin J, Perchellet JP (1973) Studies on sex differentiation in mammals. Recent Prog Horm Res 29:1–41
8. Gray LE, Jr., Wolf C, Lambright C, Mann P, Price M, Cooper RL, Ostby J (1999) Administration of potentially antiandrogenic pesticides (procymidone, linuron, iprodione, chlozolinate, p,p'-DDE, and ketoconazole) and toxic substances (dibutyl- and diethylhexyl phthalate, PCB 169, and ethane dimethane sulphonate) during sexual differentiation produces diverse profiles of reproductive malformations in the male rat. Toxicol Ind Health 15:94–118.
9. Dorfman RJ (1970) Biological activity of the antiandrogens. J Dermatol 82:4–8
10. Omezzine A, Chater S, Mauduit C, Florin A, Chuzel F, Bars R, Benahmed M (2002) Permanent increase in the expression of caspase 3 and 6 in the adult rat testis following an in utero exposure to flutamide. Submitted

11. Raff MC (1996) Size control: the regulation of cell numbers in animal development. Cell 86:173–175.
12. Strasser A, O'Connor L, Dixit VM (2000) Apoptosis signaling. Annu Rev Biochem 69:217–245
13. Kim JM, Ghosh SR, Weil AC, Zirkin BR (2001) Caspase-3 and caspase-activated deoxyribonuclease are associated with testicular germ cell apoptosis resulting from reduced intratesticular testosterone. Endocrinology 142:3809–3816.
14. Benahmed M (1996) Growth factors and cytokines in the testis. In: Male infertility: Clinical investigation, cause, evaluation and treatment. Ed.Comhaire FH. London, Chapman Hall, pp 55–96
15. Bisseling JG, Knapen MF, Goverde HJ, Mulder TP, Peters WH, Willemsen WN, Thomas CM, Steegers EA (1997) Glutathione S-transferases in human ovarian follicular fluid. Fertil Steril 68:907–911.
16. Hayes JD, Mantle TJ (1986) Use of immuno-blot techniques to discriminate between the glutathione S-transferase Yf, Yk, Ya, Yn/Yb and Yc subunits and to study their distribution in extrahepatic tissues. Evidence for three immunochemically distinct groups of transferase in the rat. Biochem J 233:779–788.
17. Ketterer B, Fraser G, Meyer DJ (1990) Nuclear glutathione transferases which detoxify irradiated DNA. Adv Exp Med Biol 264:301–310
18. Mannervik B, Danielson UH (1988) Glutathione transferases–structure and catalytic activity. CRC Crit Rev Biochem 23:283–337
19. Pickett CB, Lu AY (1989) Glutathione S-transferases: gene structure, regulation, and biological function. Annu Rev Biochem 58:743–764
20. Vos RM, Van Bladeren PJ (1990) Glutathione S-transferases in relation to their role in the biotransformation of xenobiotics. Chem Biol Interact 75:241–265
21. Peltola V, Huhtaniemi I, Ahotupa M (1992) Antioxidant enzyme activity in the maturing rat testis. J Androl 13:450–455.
22. Gu W, Hecht NB (1996) Developmental expression of glutathione peroxidase, catalase, and manganese superoxide dismutase mRNAs during spermatogenesis in the mouse. J Androl 17:256–262.
23. Rao AV, Shaha C (2000) Role of glutathione S-transferases in oxidative stress-induced male germ cell apoptosis. Free Radic Biol Med 29:1015–1027.
24. Yang Y, Cheng JZ, Singhal SS, Saini M, Pandya U, Awasthi S, Awasthi YC (2001) Role of Glutathione S-Transferases in Protection against Lipid Peroxidation. Overexpression of hGSTa2–2 in k562 cells protects against hydrogen peroxide-induced apoptosis and inhibits JNK and caspase 3 activation. J Biol Chem 276:19220–19230.

25. Benbrahim-Tallaa L, Tabone E, Mauduit C, Chuzel F, Bars R, Benahmed M (2002) In utero exposure to flutamide permanently alters glutathione S-transferase alpha expression in the adult rat testis. Submitted

3 Understanding the Mutation-Induced Activation of the Lutropin Receptor from Computer Simulation

F. Fanelli

3.1 Introduction

The activation of different classes of plasma membrane receptors regulates the activity of practically every cell of the body. The vast majority of these receptors belong to the superfamily of G protein coupled receptors (GPCRs) which, at current estimates, account for about 1% of the genes present in a mammalian genome. Dysregulation of GPCR function is associated with a growing number of human diseases.

All the GPCRs belonging to the rhodopsin subfamily share the presence of seven hydrophobic regions that form a bundle of α-helical transmembrane domains connected by alternating intracellular and extracellular hydrophilic loops. Whereas ligand binding involves the extracellular portion of the receptor, the intracellular regions mediate the interaction of the receptor with G proteins as well as other signalling and regulatory proteins.

Theoretically all proteins that comprise the signal transduction pathways of GPCRs are potential targets for mutational events that can lead to constitutive (agonist independent) signalling or inactivation and, consequently, disease. Indeed, mutations of a number of GPCRs and G proteins have been shown to cause disease in humans [1–3]. In this respect, the GPCRs that bind the glycoprotein hormones like the human chorionic gonadotropin (hCG) the luteinizing hormone (LH), the follicle-stimulating hormone (FSH) and the thyroid-stimulating hormone (TSH) are particularly prone to be sources of genetic diseases [1, 2]. In particular, activating mutations of the LH receptor (LHR) result in familial male-limited precocious puberty (FMPP), whereas, mutations that cause inactivation of this receptor result in complete pseudohermaphroditism in men and anovulation in women [1, 4].

Detailed knowledge about the molecular structure and dynamics of GPCRs is therefore likely to open new therapeutic perspectives, particularly in the genetic disease field. However, understanding the mechanism of functioning of the GPCR micromachinery has the drawback that high-resolution structural information of these membrane proteins is lacking.

During the last seven years, we have extensively used constitutively active and inactive mutants as probes for investigating the activation mechanism of several GPCRs of the rhodopsin family [5–12]. The study essentially concerned 3D model building and molecular dynamics (MD) simulations of the native forms as well as of engineered and spontaneous mutants of the α1b-adrenergic receptor (α1b-AR) and the LHR [5–7, 9–12]. The molecular models of these receptors were achieved following an ab initio approach, i.e. without using any structure of homologous proteins as templates.

Recently, Palczewski and colleagues have published the crystal structure of bovine rhodopsin determined at 2.8 Å resolution [13]. Taking advantage of this major advance in the field, natural and engineered mutants of the LHR have been also simulated on a new receptor model achieved by comparative modelling [11, 12, 14, 15].

The present work focuses on the insights gained so far into our understanding of the structural requirements that make a LHR site susceptible to activating mutations as well as of the structural peculiarities of the active and inactive LHR forms.

3.2 Methods

3.2.1 Building and Computer Simulation of Ab Initio and Homology Models of the LHR

The first molecular models of the LHR have been built following an ab initio procedure based on the integration of computational chemistry and bioinformatics tools with the results of mutational, biophysical and biochemical experiments on GPCRs [9]. The ab initio LHR model also holds the structural information as inferred from the electron micrographs of three-dimensional frog rhodopsin crystals [16], as well as from the analysis of ~500 GPCR sequences [17], and comprises the seven transmembrane helices and the connecting extracellular and intracellular loops. Comparative Molecular Dynamics (MD) simulations (by means of the program CHARMm [18]) have been performed on the wild type LHR, as well as on all the naturally occurring activating and inactivating mutations discovered thus far [4]. The strategy used has been to elaborate a unique input structure (i.e. that is the same for the wild type and the mutants, except for the mutated amino acid side chain) able to produce, upon MD simulations, divergent average arrangements for the active and inactive receptor forms [9]. The receptor structures averaged over the 200 structures collected during the last 100 ps of a 150 ps MD trajectory and minimised have been finally employed for the comparative analysis [9].

The average minimised structure of the wild type LHR achieved by ab initio modelling show a root mean square deviation (RMSD) of 4.57 Å from the rhodopsin structure [13]. RMSD has been computed by superimposing the main-chain atoms of segments 37–62, 74–99, 111–133, 152–171, 202–225, 253–276 and 286–306, representing the seven transmembrane domains of rhodopsin, with those in the homologous segments 359–384, 396–422, 440–462, 482–501, 526–549, 570–593, and 603–623 of the average minimised structure of the wild type LHR.

Very recently, a new model of the human LHR has been achieved by comparative modelling [14] (by means of the MODELLER program [19]), using the crystal structure of rhodopsin as a template [13].

The wild type and mutant structures have been energy minimised and subjected to MD simulations by following the same computational protocol as that previously used for the ab initio models [9] and the resulting average minimised structures have been finally employed for the comparative analysis.

The average minimised structures of the wild type achieved by comparative modelling diverges from the rhodopsin structure by 2.54 Å. These deviations are close to the expected values, considering the sequence identity (22.2%) between the matched segments of the LHR and rhodopsin [20].

3.3 Results and Discussion

3.3.1 Structural Features of the Activating Mutation Sites

In order to infer hypotheses on the structural features that make a receptor site susceptible to activating mutations, we have subjected to MD simulations all the spontaneously occurring activating and inactivating mutations of the LHR known so far [4, 10]. Moreover, selected activating mutation sites have been deeply investigated by extensive computer-simulated and experimental mutagenesis [11, 12, 14, 15].

The analysis of the mutant structures within both the ab initio and the homology models suggest that in the LHR, the sites susceptible to activating mutations (highlighted in green in Fig. 1) are inter-helical positions close to highly conserved polar amino acids (highlighted in purple in Fig. 1).

Both the ab initio and homology models suggest that activating mutations may cause either gain or loss or just change in the interaction performed by the native amino acid.

In some receptor sites, only selected substitutions cause constitutive activity. This is the case of L457. In fact, experimental findings suggest that only the replacements of L457 with cationic amino acids lead to constitutively active forms of the LHR [11, 12]. Computer simulations suggest that the need of a cationic amino acid in position 457 triggering constitutive activation is linked to the closeness of D578 in helix 6, that would stabilise the active state of the receptor by making a salt bridge with the cationic amino acid substituting for L457 [11]. In the case of L457R, the most active among the engineered mutants of L457, the replacing amino acid is also involved in H-bonding interactions with the

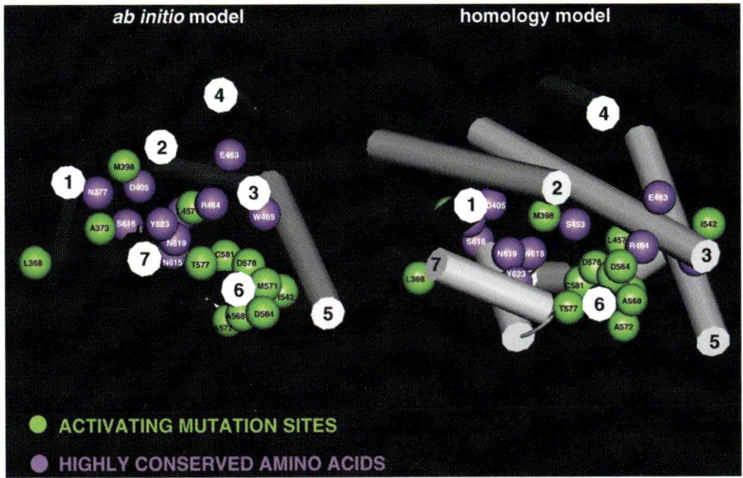

Fig. 1. Average minimised structures of the wild type LHR achieved by ab initio modelling (*left*) and comparative modelling (*right*). A cylinder representation of the helix-bundles is shown, viewed from the intracellular side in a direction almost perpendicular to the membrane surface. The spheres, centred on the β-carbon atoms of the amino acid side chains, indicate the location of the LHR sites susceptible to spontaneous activating mutations (*green spheres*) and the location of the ERW motif as well as of highly conserved amino acids (*purple spheres*)

highly conserved asparagines N615 and N619 in helix 7 [11]. Thus, gain of specific interactions characterises the L457 active mutants.

For some receptor sites, the extent of constitutive activity is independent of the amino acid substitution. This is the case of D564 and D578. As for D564, experiments have shown that substitutions of this aspartate with G, A, V, L, F, K and N, that would break or weaken a salt bridge with a putative cationic amino acid, result in constitutive activation, whereas substitution with glutamate does not [21, 22]. As for D578, experiments have shown that mutating this aspartate into nine different natural amino acids induces constitutive activation of the LHR, independently of the physico-chemical properties of the substituting amino acid, the mutation to asparagine showing a normal activity [23]. In particular, the homology model suggests that the activating mutations of D578 cause the breakage or simply a perturbation in the H-bonding interaction found in the wild type between D578 and N615 [14, 15]. Interestingly, simulations and experiments suggest that activating mutations of D578 need the integrity of the highly conserved N615 and N619 in helix 7 to be fully functional [15]. Thus, loss of charge-reinforced H-bonding interactions are predicted to be the triggers of the activation induced by mutations of D564 and D578.

In some other cases, it is possible to find quantitative relationships between the chemico-physical properties of the replacing amino acid and the extent of the constitutive activity induced by mutation [14]. This is the case of M398, that has been subjected to fifteen different amino acid substitutions. Indeed, the basal activity of the M398 mutants is inversely correlated with the size of the replacing amino acid. Consistent with this relation, molecular simulations have suggested that reducing the size of the amino acid at position 398 reduces the intramolecular interactions played by the mutated amino acid and confers to the receptor structure the features of the active forms [14]. Thus, loss of dispersive interactions could be the local perturbation triggered by activating mutations of M398.

The activating mutation sites, in spite of the structural and topological differences among them, show a structural connection with peculiar portions of the cytosolic domains like the interface between helices 3 and 6. This connection is mediated by the highly conserved amino acids in the seven-helix bundle.

3.3.2 Structural Features of the Inactive and Active LHR forms

The main differences between ab initio and homology models essentially concern the interaction pattern involving the arginine of the E/DRY/W sequence in the inactive states. In particular, according to the ab initio model, R464 interacts with the adjacent glutamate and/or with the highly conserved D405 in helix 2 [9, 10]. In contrast, according to the homology model, in the wild type and the inactive mutants, the highly conserved arginine is involved into a salt bridge with both the adjacent E463 and D564 in helix 6. Despite these differences both the ab initio and the homology models suggest that activating mutations induce the breakage or weakening of one or both the salt bridge interactions involving the highly conserved arginine in the wild type and the inactive mutants. These structural modifications are associated with the increase in solvent accessibility of selected amino acids at the cytosolic extensions of helices 3 and 6, effect that is accounted for by two different indices in the ab initio and homology models [9–12, 14, 15]. These theoretical indices have been successfully used to predict the functional behaviour of single and multiple LHR mutants [14, 15].

The theoretical models are consistent with the data implicating the cytosolic extensions of helix 5 and helix 6 as being involved in G protein activation by the LHR [12, 24].

3.4 Conclusions

The results of molecular simulations on different LHR models converge into the hypothesis that the arginine of E/DRY/W sequence is an important switch of the LHR activation. However, whether this arginine is important for the LHR activation or for G protein recognition/activation still remains unclear.

The results of this study also suggest that a structural modification at the interface between the cytosolic extensions of helix 3 and helix 6 is important in the mutation-induced LHR activation and/or G protein recognition. This hypothesis is consistent with a number of studies demonstrating that a rearrangement in the relative position of helix 3 and helix 6 is a fundamental step in GPCR activation [25–27].

The theoretical models provide insights into the structural features of the LHR sites susceptible to spontaneous activating mutations, constituting also useful tools for "in silico" prediction of the functional behaviour of LHR mutants.

References

1. Shenker A. (1995) G protein coupled receptor structure and function: the impact of disease-causing mutations. *Baillière's Clini Endocrinol Metab* **9**: 427–451.
2. Arvanitakis L, Geras-Raaka E, Gershengorn MC (1998) Constitutively Signaling G-protein coupled receptor and human disease. *Trends Endocrin Metabol* **9**:27–31.
3. Farfel Z, Bourne HR., Taroh I (1999) The expanding spectrum of G protein diseases. *New Engl J Med* **340**:1012–1019.
4. Themmen APN, Huhtaniemi IT (2000) Mutations of gonadotropins and gonadotropin receptors: elucidating the physiology and pathophysiology of pituitary-gonadal function. *Endoc Rev.* **21**:551–583.
5. Scheer A, Fanelli F, Costa T, De Benedetti P G, Cotecchia S (1996) Constitutively active mutants of the α1B-adrenergic receptor: role of highly conserved polar amino acids in receptor activation. *EMBO J.* **15**: 3566–3578.
6. Scheer A, Fanelli F, Costa T, De Benedetti PG, Cotecchia S (1997) The activation process of the α1B-adrenergic receptor: potential role of protonation and hydrophobicity of a highly conserved aspartate. *Proc Natl Acad Sci USA* **94**: 808–813.
7. Fanelli F, Menziani MC, Scheer A, Cotecchia S, De Benedetti PG (1999) Theoretical study on the electrostatically driven step of receptor-G protein recognition. *PROTEINS: Strucure, Function and Genetics*, **37**: 145–156.
8. Fanelli F, Barbier P, Zanchetta D, De Benedetti PG, Chini B (1999) Activation Mechanism of Human Oxytocin Receptor: A Combined Study of Experimental and Computer-Simulated Mutagenesis. *Mol. Pharmacol.* **56**:214–225.
9. Fanelli F (2000) Theoretical study on mutation-induced activation of the luteinizing hormone receptor. *J. Mol. Biol.*, **296**: 1337–1355.
10. Latronico AC, Shinozaki H, Guerra G Jr, Pereira MAA, Helena S, Marini VL, Baptista MTM, Arnhold IJP, Fanelli F, Mendonca BB, Segaloff DL (2000) Gonadotropin-independent precocious puberty due to luteinizing hormone receptor mutations in brasilian boys: a novel constitutively activating mutation in the first transmembrane helix. *J Clini Endocrin Metabol* **85**: 4799–4805.
11. Shinozaki H, Fanelli F, Liu X, Butterbrodt J, Nakamura K, Segaloff DL (2001) Pielotropic effects of substitutions of a highly conserved leucine in transmembrane helix III of the human lutropin/choriogonadotropin receptor with respect to constitutive activation and hormone responsiveness. *Mol. Endocrinol.* **15**: 972–984.
12. Ascoli M, Fanelli F, Segaloff DL The lutropin/choriogonadotropin receptor, a 2001 perspective *Endocr. Rev.*, in press.

13. Palczewski K, Kumasaka T, Hori T, Behnke CA, Motoshima H, Fox BA, LeTrong I, Teller DC, Okada T, Stenkamp RE, Yamamoto M, Miyano M (2000) Crystal structure of rhodopsin: a G protein-coupled receptor. *Science* **289**:739–745.

14. Fanelli F, Verhoef-Post M, Timmerman M, Zeilemaker A, van Marle A, Martens JWM, and Themmen APN, manuscript in preparation.

15. Angelova K, Fanelli F, Puett D. Engineered and Simulated Mutations in Transmembrane Helices 6 and 7 of the Lutropin Receptor: A Model for Constitutive and Ligand-mediated Receptor Activation, submitted for publication.

16. Unger VM, Hargrave PA, Baldwin JM, Schertler GF (1997). Arrangement of rhodopsin transmembrane α-helices. *Nature*, **389**: 203–206.

17. Baldwin JM, Schertler GF, Unger VM (1997). An alpha-carbon atom template for the transmembrane helices in the rhodopsin family of G-protein-coupled receptors. *J Mol. Biol.*, **272**:144–164.

18. Brooks BR, Bruccoleri RE, Olafson BD, States DJ, Swaminathan S, Karplus M (1983). Charmm: a program for macromolecular energy, minimization and dynamics calculations. *J. Comput. Chem.*, **4**:187–217.

19. Sali A, Blundell TL (1993) Comparative protein modeling by satisfaction of spatial restraints. *J Mol. Biol.* **234**: 779–815.

20. Chothia C. Lesk AM (1986) The relation between the divergence of sequence and structure in proteins *Embo J.*, **5**:823–6.

21. Schulz A, Schöneberg T, Paschke R, Schultz G, Gudermann T (1999)). Role of the third intracellular loop for the activation of gonadotropin receptors. *Mol. Endocrinol.*, **13**:181–190.

22. Kosugi S, Mori T, Shenker A (1998) An anionic residue at position 564 is important for maintaining the inactive conformation of the human lutropin/choriogonadotropin receptor. *Mol. Pharmacol.*, **53**: 894–901

23. Kosugi S, Mori T, Shenker A (1996) The role of Asp578 in maintaining the inactive conformation of the human lutropin/choriogonadotropin receptor. *J. Biol. Chem.*, **271**: 31813–31817.

24. Abell AN, McCormick J, Segaloff DJ (1998) Certain activating mutations within helix 6 of the human luteinizing hormone receptor may be explained by alterations that allow transmembrane regions to activate Gs. *Mol. Endocrinol.* **12**:1857–1869.

25. Farrens DL, Altenbach C. Yang K, Hubbell WL, Khorana HG (1996) Requirement of rigid-body motion of transmembrane helices for light activation of rhodopsin. *Science* **274**: 768–770.

26. Sheikh SP, Zvyaga TA, Lichtarge O, Sakmar TP, Bourne HB (1996) Rhodopsin activation blocked by metal-ion-binding sites linking transmembrane helices C and F. *Nature* **383**: 347–350 .

27. Gether U (2000) Uncovering molecular mechanisms involved in activation
    of G protein-coupled receptors. *Endocr. Rev.* **21**: 90–113.

4 Sex-Specific Differences in the Control of Mammalian Gametogenesis: Vive la Difference!

D.J. Wolgemuth

4.1 Introduction

The notion that the highly differentiated mammalian gametes would
have gamete-specific genes that are important for their differentiation
and function is almost self-evident. The structural components of these
specialized cells, such as proteins in the acrosome, flagellum, and zona
pellucida would be expected to and indeed do exhibit sexually dimorphic expression and function. This class of sex-specific genes is ex-
cluded from the following discussion. Rather, we will explore the roles
of genes that by virtue of their common expression in both oocytes and
spermatocytes or their conserved function in gametes across species
might be expected to be important to germ cell function in mammals –
yet have proven to defy our best predictions!

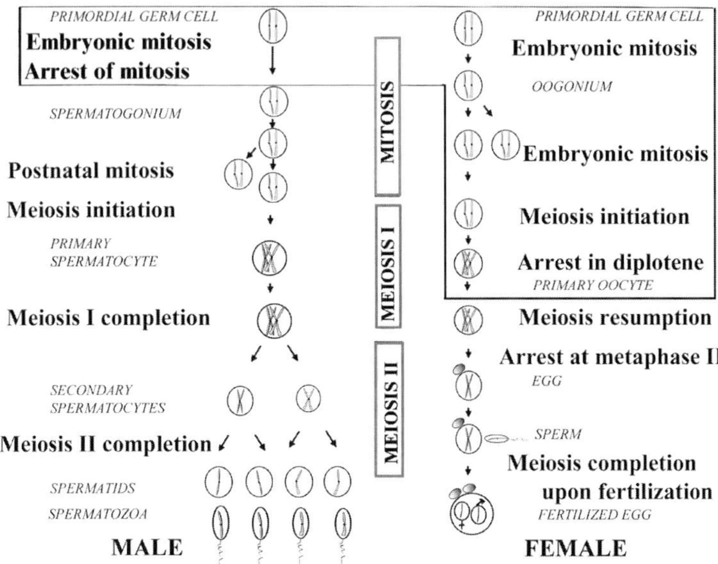

Fig. 1. Cartoon of key stages of mammalian gametogenesis. The state of the mitotic and meiotic cell cycles are noted and differences between male and female gametogenesis is highlighted. The stages included within the *box* occur during embryonic development in most mammals. (Adapted from Alberts et al 1983 and Wolgemuth 1995)

4.1.1 Overview of Mammalian Gametogenesis

Mammalian gametogenesis in both sexes involves a highly orchestrated series of mitotic proliferations, meiotic recombination followed by reduction divisions, and subsequent differentiation to produce the highly specialized germ cells, the egg and the sperm [reviewed in (Bellve et al. 1977; Setchell 1982; Bachvarova 1985; Schultz 1986; Eddy et al. 1993)]. Although these events occur during both male and female germ cell development in mammals, the temporal pattern of their progression is quite different (Fig. 1). In both sexes in mice, primordial germ cells colonize the sexually indifferent genital ridge between the 11th and 12th day of fetal life and become incorporated into the sex cords. At this time they enter a non-proliferative growth phase and are referred to as gonocytes. An immediate difference is observed between fetal male and female gonad development, in that oogonia differentiate and enter into meiosis by day 12–13. In contrast, spermatogonia only begin to differentiate in the first week after birth (Nebel et al. 1961). The type A spermatogonium is the stem cell, producing more type A cells or giving rise to type B spermatogonia, which differentiate into pre-leptotene spermatocytes and enter prophase.

Meiotic prophase begins at approximately post-natal day 8 in the male mouse (the exact timing varies between strains), lasts 1 week and is followed by two reduction divisions that produce haploid spermatids. The round (early) spermatid first appears at post-natal day 18 and undergoes a series of unique morphological transformations during its differentiation into a spermatozoan. Spermiogenesis has been divided into 16 stages based on changes in the acrosome and the nucleus (Oakberg 1956a; Russel et al. 1990). In addition to acrosome formation and nuclear condensation, this period of morphogenesis includes the formation of the flagellum and the elimination of excess cytoplasm as the residual body. In the mouse, the entire process from spermatogonia to fully differentiated spermatozoa is completed in approximately 35 days and a new round is initiated approximately every 12 days (Oakberg 1956a). The relative synchrony in the developmental progression of spermatogenesis in the prepuberal animal provides a useful approach for assigning the expression of specific genes to particular cell types. That is, testis at early post-natal stages will lack more advanced cell types (Nebel et al. 1961).

Furthermore, the constant and synchronous nature of the spermatogenic process results in specific patterns of tubule organization and cellular associations during germ cell differentiation, such that cells at particular stages of differentiation will be associated with one another at a given site in the tubule. These associations are a consequence of the fact that initiation of a new round of spermatogenesis occurs before preceding ones have finished. In mouse, these associations have been classified into 12 stages of cycling of the seminiferous epithelium (Oakberg 1956a).

In contrast, female mammalian germ cells continue to undergo mitotic divisions after entering the embryonic gonad and, in most species, enter into meiosis, arresting at diplotene of meiosis I. At birth, these "resting" oocytes are found in primordial follicles, surrounded by a single layer of granulosa cells. Puberty is marked by the recruitment of a pool of oocytes into a growth period in response to cyclic variations in gonadotrophins. During this growth period, the oocyte increases in size but remains arrested in prophase of meiosis I. Concomitantly, the number of granulosa cells surrounding the oocyte increases. After completion of this growth and proliferative phase to form the mature follicle, the oocyte is stimulated to resume meiosis. Meiosis I is completed and the ovum is ovulated while arrested in metaphase of meiosis II, awaiting fertilization to complete the second meiotic division.

The somatic compartment of the gonads is also distinct between the sexes, particularly with respect to their cellular proliferation in the adult. Both Sertoli cells and interstitial cells are mitotically most active in the fetal and immature testis. However in the adult animal, Sertoli cells undergo little or no proliferation. In contrast, ovarian follicle cells, which correspond to Sertoli cells, undergo considerable cell division as selected follicles grow before ovulation.

4.1.2 Focus on Cell Cycle Regulation During Mitosis and Meiosis

Understanding the genetic program controlling the mitotic and meiotic divisions of the germ line will provide insight into understanding infertility and new directions for contraception. This is of particular relevance to the male in which new developments in contraception have been lagging for the last hundred years! Male and female germ cells have aspects of cell cycle regulation that are similar between the two lineages, including the mitotic proliferative stage, entry into meiosis, completion of a reductive division, and entry into a quiescent state awaiting fertilization. However, the timing of these events and indeed even the stage of development at which these events occur differ in the two sexes (Fig. 1; reviewed in Wolgemuth et al. 1995). As noted above, in most mammals, female germ cells enter meiosis during fetal development, whereas this is a post-natal event in the male. Once the male germ cell has entered meiosis, the process continues without interruption to produce haploid spermatids. In contrast, the oocyte is arrested in the diplotene stage of meiotic prophase I, where it can remain for months or years. Following a growth period, the oocyte resumes meiosis, only to be arrested a second time, at metaphase II. Fertilization then triggers the completion of meiosis and extrusion of the second polar body.

4.2 Examples of Genes That Are Differentially Expressed and Have Distinct Functions During Male and Female Meiosis

4.2.1 Focus on the A-Type Cyclins

Several years ago, our laboratory began to focus on the role of the cyclins in the control of mitosis and meiosis during gametogenesis in the mouse model. Our studies on the A-type cyclins revealed that there are two distinct cyclin A genes in mammals, cyclin A1 and A2. They share 44% identity at the overall amino acid level but share a much higher level of identity (84%) within the two highly conserved cyclin boxes (Ravnik and Wolgemuth 1996; Sweeney et al. 1996). Two A-type cyclin genes have now been documented in human and frog as well (Howe et al. 1995; Yang et al. 1997).

In the adult mouse, Northern blot hybridization analysis revealed that expression of cyclin A1 was restricted to the testis, specifically to germ cells. In situ hybridization analysis and immunohistochemistry were used to localize their expression to specific testicular cells. The levels of cyclin A1 mRNA (Sweeney et al. 1996; Liu et al. 1998) and protein (Liu et al. 1998; Ravnik and Wolgemuth 1999) rise dramatically in late pachytene spermatocytes and become undetectable soon after completion of the first meiotic division. At both the RNA and protein levels, the predominant sites of cyclin A2 expression in the adult testis are strikingly different. Cyclin A2 is expressed in the mitotic germ line stem cells, the spermatogonia, and in preleptotene spermatocytes, cells in which premeiotic DNA synthesis occurs (Ravnik and Wolgemuth 1996; Ravnik and Wolgemuth 1999). Cyclin A2 expression is also detected in Leydig cells (Ge and Hardy 1997). The concurrent localization of mRNA and protein for both of the A-type cyclins further suggested that both are regulated primarily at the level of transcription in the testis. The observed cellular specificity of cyclin A2 expression is consistent with its function during mitosis in the stem cell stage of this lineage, while the restricted preleptotene stage localization suggests that cyclin A2

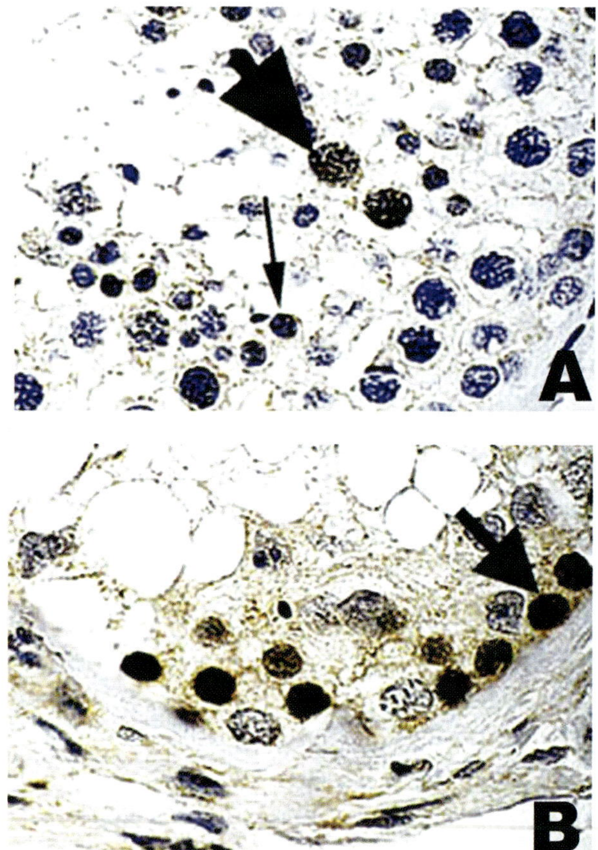

Fig. 2A, B. Immunohistochemical localization of cyclin A1 and cyclin A2 in histological sections of human testes. *Large arrows* indicate pachytene spermatocytes in **A** and pre-leptotene spermatocytes in **B**. The *thin arrow* in **A** denotes a spermatid

may function in G1/S or S but not in the meiotic divisions. We have recently extended our analysis to the human testis as well. Illustrated in Fig. 2 is the localization of cyclin A1 protein in human testes to pachytene and diplotene spermatocytes and cyclin A2 in spermatogonia and in cells that appear to be pre-leptotene spermatocytes.

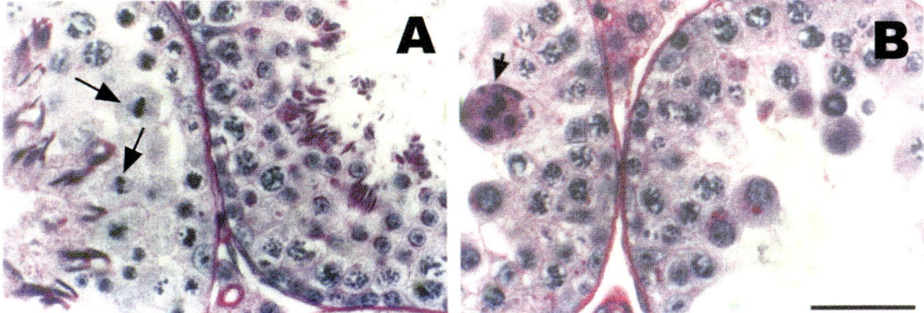

Fig. 3A, B. Spermatogenesis is disrupted in cyclin A1-deficient testes. Normal testis (**A**) with spermatocytes in the first meiotic division (*arrows*). Cyclin A1-deficient testis (**B**) lacking spermatids and containing giant cells. (Adapted from Liu et al 1998)

In contrast, no cyclin A1 mRNA was detected in mouse ovaries or oocytes by Northern or in situ hybridization analysis (Liao et al., in preparation). However, both somatic and germ cells of the adult ovary express cyclin A2 mRNA and protein. The different expression patterns suggest distinct functions for cyclin A1 and cyclin A2 in the somatic and germinal lineages, which also differ between the male and female.

Cyclin A2 is expressed ubiquitously in cultured cells and in a broad variety of tissues in the adult mouse and during embryogenesis, e.g. (Ravnik and Wolgemuth 1996; Sweeney et al. 1996). Perhaps not surprisingly, targeted mutagenesis of the murine cyclin A2 gene resulted in early embryonic lethality, apparently around the peri-implantation stage (Murphy et al. 1997). This embryonic lethality has obviated understanding the role of cyclin A2 in other aspects of mammalian development, including the germ line.

The strikingly restricted expression of cyclin A1 led us to hypothesize that its primary site of function is in the male germ line, specifically at the first meiotic division. To test this hypothesis, we generated cyclin A1-deficient mice by targeted mutagenesis of the cyclin A1 gene (Liu et al. 1998). Cyclin A1-deficient males are sterile due to a block of spermatogenesis before the first meiotic division (Fig. 3), whereas females are normal. Meiosis arrest in males lacking cyclin A1 was associated with increased germ cell apoptosis and desynapsis abnormalities (Liu et al.

1998). There is a striking reduction in the activation of MPF kinase at the end of meiotic prophase, although both Cdk1 and cyclin B proteins were present (Liu et al. 2000). Cyclin A1 is therefore essential for spermatocyte passage into the first meiotic division in male mice, a function that cannot be complemented by the concurrently expressed B-type cyclins.

We explored the possibility that a cyclin A1-dependent process dictates the activation of MPF (Liu et al. 1998). First, we asked if the expression of the B-type cyclins that comprise MPF was retained in cyclin A1-deficient spermatocytes (Liu et al. 2000). Both cyclin B1 and B2 proteins were readily detected, although their associated kinases were kept at inactive states. We then turned to an in vitro short-term culture system developed by Handel and colleagues (Wiltshire et al. 1995) to ask whether okadaic acid treatment of pachytene-diplotene spermatocytes in cyclin A1-deficient testes could drive the cells into meiosis I and activate MPF activity. Indeed, okadaic acid treatment of cyclin A1-deficient spermatocytes restored MPF activity and induced entry into M phase. Overtly normally condensed chromosome bivalents were formed and hyperphosphorylation of Cdc25 proteins was observed (Liu et al. 2000). In this system treatment of pachytene spermatocytes with the protein phosphatase type-1 and –2A inhibitor okadaic acid can induce premature chromosome condensation and entry into the first meiotic division.

As noted above, the early embryonic lethality of the cyclin A2 null mutation (Murphy et al. 1997; Winston et al. 2000) obviates a direct test of its function in either the male or female germ line. To examine the function of cyclin A2 during oogenesis and in pre-meiotic spermatogenesis, it would be of interest to consider the use of conditional mutagenesis. One such approach would involve the generation of transgenic mice expressing the Cre recombinase uniquely in spermatogonia and/or preleptotene spermatocytes, under the direction of a promoter specific to these cells. These animals would then be crossed to mice carrying the cyclin A2 gene into which loxP sites have been introduced (floxed cyclin A2). Excision of portions of the cyclin A2 gene between the loxP sites would result in a mutant cyclin A2 gene, but only in spermatogonia or preleptotene spermatocytes.

The critical missing link in this approach is the lack of well-characterized, spermatogonia-specific promoters. The Cre-lox strategies using oocyte-specific promoters to drive Cre recombinase might be fruitful to address the role of cyclin A2 in oocyte mitosis and especially, meiosis. Promoters for oocyte-specific genes such as zona pellucida 3 have been well-characterized in transgenic animals and have been recently applied to the Cre-lox system as well (Lewandoski et al. 1997).

Alternatively, the recent application of double-stranded RNAs (RNAi) to interfere with gene expression in oocytes might also permit a direct test of the cyclin A2 protein in the resumption of meiosis (Svoboda et al. 2000). In this approach, double stranded RNAs for the *c-mos* proto-oncogene were shown to inhibit the translation of *c-mos* mRNA in a time and concentration-dependent manner. Importantly, this inhibition resulted in parthenogenetic activation of the oocytes, similar to the phenotype observed in *c-mos* knockout mouse oocytes (Colledge et al. 1994; Hashimoto et al. 1994).

4.3 Other Non-Structural Genes with Sex-Specific Expression and/or Function

4.3.1 *c-mos* Proto-oncogene

In vivo characterization of the expression of the proto-oncogene *c-mos* revealed that the predominant sites of expression were the testis and ovary. In a series of detailed studies on the distribution of *c-mos* mRNA (Goldman et al. 1987; Mutter et al. 1987; Propst et al. 1987; Mutter et al. 1988), two different sized transcripts were detected in testis and ovary, of 1.7 and 1.4 kb in size respectively. In situ hybridization experiments revealed that in adult mouse ovaries, the predominant if not exclusive site of expression was growing oocytes (Mutter et al. 1987). In the testis, *c-mos* was most abundant in cells after they had entered the haploid stage of spermatogenesis. Thus, function of this proto-oncogene at in both male and female germ cells was predicted, although possibly at different stages.

An important function for *c-mos* in oocyte function has been shown by antisense oligonucleotide inhibition of expression (O'Keefe et al. 1989; Paules et al. 1989), targeted gene knockouts (Colledge et al. 1994; Hashimoto et al. 1994), and the RNAi experiments referred to above. However, no defects in fertility were observed in the male mice homozygous for a null mutation in *c-mos*. It thus appears that while *c-mos* is quite restricted in its expression in adult mouse tissues to the male and female germ lines, it is essential only for proper oogenesis.

4.3.2 DNA Mismatch Repair Gene *Pms2*

The human *PMS2* gene has been identified as one of the putative mammalian homologues of the bacterial DNA mismatch repair gene *mutL* and known to be associated with hereditary nonpolyposis colorectal cancer (Bronner et al. 1994). One characteristic of the tumors is frequent alteration in the length of microsatellite DNA sequences (Aaltonen et al. 1993). Studies in yeast showed that DNA mismatch repair enzymes also function during genetic recombination in meiosis (Alani et al. 1994). It was therefore hypothesized that a deficiency in mismatch repair enzymes could have consequences in the germline (Baker et al. 1995). Indeed, targeted disruption of the mouse *Pms2* gene resulted in sterility in the male but curiously not the female germ line (Baker et al. 1995). The males produced only abnormal spermatozoa and analysis of axial element and synaptonemal complex formation during meiotic prophase indicated abnormalities in chromosome synapsis. In contrast, female mice deficient for *Pms2* are fully fertile, with normal pregnancy rates and litter sizes. Until it is known whether in fact *Pms2* is expressed in the germ line of both male and females, it cannot be concluded that there are male-specific requirements for *Pms2* during meiosis as opposed to male-specific expression of *Pms2*. Nonetheless, a male-specific function was observed.

4.3.3 Retinoic Acid Receptor Alpha

It has been recognized for many years that retinoids, a class of naturally-occurring and synthetic compounds that are structurally related to vitamin A are required for various aspects of normal reproduction. In particular, vitamin A-deficiency in male rats has been shown to result in sterility due to abnormalities in germ cell development; although female mice are also defective in reproduction, defects in female germ cell development are not documented.

Further support for a direct role of retinoid signaling in male but not female gametogenesis is derived from the results of ablation of one of the nuclear receptors that transduce, at least in part, the signaling from the retinoid ligands. There are six groups of retinoid receptors, which are members of the steroid hormone superfamily of nuclear receptors [rev in (Packer and Wolgemuth 1999)]. They are the retinoic acid receptors (RAR) and the retinoid-X receptors (RXR), each of which has three isoforms, alpha, beta and gamma. Gene targeting of the *RARα*·gene revealed relatively few developmental abnormalities, which was somewhat unexpected given its broad distribution of expression and the known role of retinoic acid in embryonic development. Although initially described as exhibiting profound perinatal lethality (Lufkin et al. 1993), it is now known that rearing the neonates in a pathogen-free environment eliminates this aspect of the phenotype. Various explanations have been proposed for the lack of perturbation of development in the absence of *RARα*, including potential redundancy of function among the receptors. Support for this notion can be drawn from the quite profound developmental abnormalities observed when compound null alleles for the RAR's and RXR's are made in mice. For example, mice that are doubly mutant for *RARα-β2* are embryonic lethal and exhibit profound abnormalities in many organ systems (Mendelsohn et al. 1994). A notable exception to the mild phenotype in the single *RARα*-mutant mice was the observation of male sterility (Lufkin et al. 1993). Male homozygous for *RARα*-null mutant alleles are infertile and exhibit profound disruption of spermatogenesis. The epididymis contains few and abnormal germ cells and the tubules are highly disrupted with regard to the usual precise cellular associations exhibited by adult mouse testis (Oakberg 1956b; Russel et al. 1990). The overall disruption of spermatogenesis has been noted as reminiscent of the abnormalities observed in vitamin A- deficiency (Lufkin et al. 1993; Kastner et al. 1996), although specific effects on discrete stages of spermatogenesis remains to be elucidated between the two models. Furthermore, clear separation of primary versus secondary effects must be defined.

While the male sterility phenotype is profound and highly penetrant, female mice that are deficient for *RARα* are fertile (Lufkin et al. 1993; our unpublished observations). There may exist subtle changes in the female germ line, but to date, no obvious differences in *RARα*-deficient females have been reported. *RARα* has been reported to be expressed in both the somatic and germinal compartments in testicular tubules across a broad range of spermatogenic development reviewed in e.g., Packer and Wolgemuth 1999). Although much less is known about the expression of the RARs and RXRs in the female gonad, a direct requirement for *RAR*α in oogenesis is unlikely given the lack of an effect during oogenesis in *RAR*α null animals. However, Morita and Tilly (1999) have suggested that retinoic acid mediates fetal ovarian germ cell mitosis and prevents apoptosis and that these effects are mediated through *RAR*α. They document expression of *RAR*α in ovarian germ cells at stages comparable to a subset of the expression of expression of *RAR*α in male germ cells as well. Nonetheless, the majority of current evidence would suggest sex-specific differences in the requirement for retinoids, or at least *RAR*α, in male versus female gametogenesis.

Acknowledgements. This work was supported in part by grants from the NIH, R01 HD34915 and P01 DK54057. Appreciation is extended to current and former members of the Wolgemuth laboratory whose data and insight have provided the basis for many of the topics presented in this brief chapter. In particular, thanks are extended to Erika Laurion for help in preparation of this manuscript.

References

Aaltonen LA, Peltomaki P, Leach FS, Sistonen P, Pylkkanen L, Mecklin JP, Jarvinen H, Powell SM, Jen J and Hamilton SR (1993) Clues to the pathogenesis of familial colorectal cancer. Science 260: 812–6.

Albert B, Bray D, Lewis J, Raff M, Roberts K and Watson JD (1983) Molecular Biology of The Cell. Garland Publishing, Inc.

Alani E, Reenan RA and Kolodner RD (1994) Interaction between mismatch repair and genetic recombination in Saccharomyces cerevisiae. Genetics 137: 19–39.

Bachvarova R (1985) Gene expression during oogenesis and oocyte development in mammals. In: Developmental Biology. Eds. L. W. Browder. New York, pp 453–524.

Baker SM, Bronner CE, Zhang L, Plug AW, Robatzek M, Warren G, Elliott EA, Yu J, Ashley T and Arnheim N (1995) Male mice defective in the DNA mismatch repair gene PMS2 exhibit abnormal chromosome synapsis in meiosis. Cell 82: 309–19.

Bellve AR, Cavicchia JC, Millette CF, O'Brien DA, Bhatnagar YM and Dym M (1977) Spermatogenic cells of the prepuberal mouse. Isolation and morphological characterization. J Cell Biol 741: 68–85

Bronner CE, Baker SM, Morrison PT, Warren G, Smith LG, Lescoe MK, Kane M, Earabino C, Lipford J and Lindblom A (1994) Mutation in the DNA mismatch repair gene homologue hMLH1 is associated with hereditary non-polyposis colon cancer. Nature 368: 258–61.

Colledge WH, Carlton MB, Udy GB and Evans MJ (1994) Disruption of c-mos causes parthenogenetic development of unfertilized mouse eggs. Nature 370: 65–8

Eddy EM, Welch JE and O'Brian DA (1993) Gene expression during spermatogenesis. In: Mol Biol of the Reprod Syst. Eds. D. d. Kretser. San Diego, pp 181–232

Ge RS and Hardy MP (1997) Decreased cyclin A2 and increased cyclin G1 levels coincide with loss of proliferative capacity in rat Leydig cells during pubertal development. Endocrinology 138: 3719–3726

Goldman DS, Kiessling AA, Millette CF and Cooper GM (1987) Expression of c-mos RNA in germ cells of male and female mice. Proc Natl Acad Sci USA 84: 4509–4513

Hashimoto N, Watanabe N, Furuta Y, Tamemoto H, Sagata N, Yokoyama M, Okazaki K, Nagayoshi M, Takeda N and Ikawa Y (1994) Parthenogenetic activation of oocytes in c-mos-deficient mice. Nature 370: 68–71

Howe JA, Howell M, Hunt T and Newport JW (1995) Identification of a developmental timer regulating the stability of embryonic cyclin A and a new somatic A-type cyclin at gastrulation. Genes Dev 9: 1164–76

Kastner P, Mark M, Leid M, Gansmuller A, Chin W, Grondona JM, Decimo D, Krezel W, Dierich A and Chambon P (1996) Abnormal spermatogenesis in RXR beta mutant mice. Genes Dev 10: 80–92

Lewandoski M, Wassarman KM and Martin GR (1997) Zp3-cre, a transgenic mouse line for the activation or inactivation of loxP-flanked target genes specifically in the female germ line. Curr Biol 72: 148–51

Liao C, Ravnik S, Zhang Q, Muhlrad S and Wolgemuth D (In preparation) Differential Expression of the A-type Cyclins during Cell Cycles in the Mouse Ovary.

Liu D, Liao C and Wolgemuth DJ (2000) A Role for Cyclin A1 in the Activation of MPF and G2-M Transition during Meiosis of Male Germ Cells in Mice. Dev Biol 224: 388–400

Liu D, Matzuk MM, Sung WK, Guo Q, Wang P and Wolgemuth DJ (1998) Cyclin A1 is required for meiosis in the male mouse. Nat Genet 20: 377–380

Lufkin T, Lohnes D, Mark M, Dierich A, Gorry P, Gaub MP, LeMeur M and Chambon P (1993) High postnatal lethality and testis degeneration in retinoic acid receptor alpha mutant mice. Proc Natl Acad Sci U S A 90: 7225–7229

Mendelsohn C, Lohnes D, Decimo D, Lufkin T, LeMeur M, Chambon P and Mark M (1994) Function of the retinoic acid receptors (RARs) during development (II). Multiple abnormalities at various stages of organogenesis in RAR double mutants. Development 120: 2749–2771

Morita Y and Tilly JL (1999) Segregation of retinoic acid effects on fetal ovarian germ cell mitosis versus apoptosis by requirement for new macromolecular synthesis. Endocrinology 140: 2696–2703

Murphy M, Stinnakre MG, Senamaud-Beaufort C, Winston NJ, Sweeney C, Kubelka M, Carrington M, Brechot C and Sobczak-Thepot J (1997) Delayed early embryonic lethality following disruption of the murine cyclin A2 gene [published erratum appeared in Nat Genet 1999 Dec;23(4):481]. Nat Genet 15: 83–86

Mutter GL, Grills GS and Wolgemuth DJ (1988) Evidence for the involvement of the proto-oncogene c-mos in mammalian meiotic maturation and possibly very early embryogenesis. Embo J 7: 683–689

Mutter GL, Stacey A and Wolgemuth DJ (1987) Differential expression in murine somatic and germinal tissues of transcripts homologous to an abundant embryonal-carcinoma-cell mRNA. Differentiation 34: 126–130

Nebel BR, Amarosa AP and Hackett EA (1961) Calendar of gametogenic development in the prepubertal male mouse. Science 134: 832–833

Oakberg EF (1956a) Duration of spermatogenesis in the mouse and timing of stages of the cycle of the seminiferous epithelium. Am J Anat 99: 507–516

Oakberg EF (1956b) A description of spermiogenesis in the mouse and its use in analysis of the cycle of the seminiferous epithelium and germ cell renewal. Am J Anat 99: 391–409

O'Keefe SJ, Wolfes H, Kiessling AA and Cooper GM (1989) Microinjection of antisense c-mos oligonucleotides prevents meiosis II in the maturing mouse egg. Proc Natl Acad Sci U S A 86: 7038–7042.

Packer AI and Wolgemuth DJ (1999) Genetic and Molecular Approaches to Understanding the Role of Retinoids in Mammalian Spermatogenesis. Handbook of Experimental Pharmacology 139: 347–368

Paules RS, Buccione R, Moschel RC, Vande Woude GF and Eppig JJ (1989) Mouse Mos protooncogene product is present and functions during oogenesis. Proc Natl Acad Sci U S A 86: 5395–5399.

Propst F, Rosenberg MP, Iyer A, Kaul K and Vande Woude GF (1987) c-mos proto-oncogene RNA transcripts in mouse tissues: structural features, developmental regulation, and localization in specific cell types. Mol Cell Biol 7: 1629–1637.

Ravnik SE and Wolgemuth DJ (1996) The developmentally restricted pattern of expression in the male germ line of a murine cyclin A, cyclin A2, suggests roles in both mitotic and meiotic cell cycles. Dev Biol 173: 69–78

Ravnik SE and Wolgemuth DJ (1999) Regulation of meiosis during mammalian spermatogenesis: the A-type cyclins and their associated cyclin-dependent kinases are differentially expressed in the germ-cell lineage. Dev Biol 207: 408–418

Russel LD, Ettlin R, Sinha Hikim AP and Clegg ED (1990) Histological and Histopathological Evaluation of the Testis. Cache River Press.

Schultz RM (1986) Molecular aspects of mammalian oocytes growth and maturation. In: Experimental Approaches to Mammalian Embryonic Development. Eds. J. R. a. R. A. Pedersen. New York, Cambridge University Press, pp 195–237

Setchell BP (1982) The flow and composition of lymph from the testes of pigs with some observations on the effect of raised venous pressure. Comp Bioch Physiol A 73: 201–205

Svoboda P, Stein P, Hayashi H and Schultz RM (2000) Selective reduction of dormant maternal mRNAs in mouse oocytes by RNA interference. Development 127: 4147–4156.

Sweeney C, Murphy M, Kubelka M, Ravnik SE, Hawkins CF, Wolgemuth DJ and Carrington M (1996) A distinct cyclin A is expressed in germ cells in the mouse. Development 122: 53–64

Wiltshire T, Park C, Caldwell KA and Handel MA (1995) Induced premature G2/M-phase transition in pachytene spermatocytes includes events unique to meiosis. Dev Biol 169: 557–567

Winston N, Bourgain-Guglielmetti F, Ciemerych MA, Kubiak JZ, Senamaud-Beaufort C, Carrington M, Brechot C and Sobczak-Thepot J (2000) Early development of mouse embryos null mutant for the cyclin A2 gene occurs in the absence of maternally derived cyclin A2 gene products. Dev Biol 223: 139–153.

Wolgemuth DJ, Rhee K, Wu S and Ravnik SE (1995) Genetic control of mitosis, meiosis and cellular differentiation during mammalian spermatogenesis. Reprod Fertil Dev 7: 669–683

Yang R, Morosetti R and Koeffler HP (1997) Characterization of a second human cyclin A that is highly expressed in testis and in several leukemic cell lines. Cancer Res 57: 913–920

5 Cloning and Characterization of Male Germ-Cell-Specific Genes

H. Tanaka, M. Nozaki, K. Yomogida, Y. Nishimune

5.1 Introduction

In most multicellular organisms, fertilized eggs differentiate into somatic and germ cells. These cells become separated during the early developmental stages and have quite different roles. Germ cells maintain species continuity, whereas somatic cells ensure the constitution and activity of the individual. In other words, somatic cells help the germ cells to ensure survival and continuity of the species. Thus, germ cells play a fundamental role in multi-cellular organisms.

Two kinds of germ cells, those from the sperm and egg, are fertilized, and the haploid genomes fuse to produce the following generation, which has the same amount of genomic material as the parental cells. This system has two contradictory arms: a conservative mechanism to maintain the species and an evolutionary mechanism that allows the organisms to adapt to complex environments through meiotic recombination and random dysjunction of chromosomes. While recombination facilitates genetic diversity, precise genome-copy transfer is a prerequisite for germ cell differentiation. Thus, the study of germ cell differentiation is important to understand the evolutionary strategies of multicellular organisms, and the balancing positive and negative forces that influence species diversity on earth.

The unique differentiation mechanisms employed by multicellular organisms suggest the existence of germ-cell-specific molecules. The most straightforward strategy to elucidate differentiation systems is to identify and characterize differentiation-specific molecules and their associated genes in germ cells. In various mammals, male germ cell differentiation occurs actively and continuously in the testis after puberty, and sperm are produced throughout adulthood (Russell et al., 1990). Male germ cell differentiation from spermatogonial stem cells into sperm is completed in seminiferous tubules under the complex regulation of many different molecules (Lele and Wolgemuth, 1998), including hormones and growth factors. It takes approximately 1 month in mice and 2 months in humans for the completion of stem cell proliferation and differentiation, meiosis, generation of haploid germ cells, and morphogenesis of the developing sperm. Many dramatic morphological changes occur during spermatogenesis, especially in haploid spermatids after meiotic division. Mature sperm need to travel a long way to fertilize an egg. The round spermatids undergo marked morphological changes to become sperm during haploid germ cell differentiation, or spermiogenesis; the nucleus is compactly shaped, the mitochondria are re-arranged, the flagellum is developed and the acrosome is generated (Bellve and O'Brien 1983). During this period of differentiation and development, which takes about 5–6 weeks in humans (Heller and Clermont 1963; Clermont 1963) or 2–3 weeks in mice (Oakberg 1956), haploid germ cells do not divide, but morphogenesis occurs, indicating that some regulatory mechanism arrests the cell cycle. Comprehensive analysis of haploid germ-cell-specific genes showed that a large number of specific molecules were involved in spermiogenesis. Further study is needed to clarify the relationships between specific molecules and their morphological and functional roles in spermiogenesis. In this report, we describe our recent findings regarding germ-cell-specific genes and gene products, with particular emphasis on haploid germ-cell-specific genes, and we discuss the relevance of our approaches to the study of germ cell differentiation mechanisms.

5.2 Identification of Germ-Cell-Specific Genes

The identification and isolation of germ-cell-specific molecules has been achieved using immunological, biochemical and molecular biological techniques. Many novel molecules have been isolated and characterized using monoclonal or specific polyclonal antibodies, and via cDNA cloning techniques (Tanaka et al. 1998). Recent progress in molecular biology has stimulated investigations of complex biological processes. Microarray techniques and the computer-assisted identification of specific genes are powerful methods for the isolation of genes that are specifically expressed in testes (Olesen et al. 2001). The isolation of cDNA and the characterization of encoded proteins that are specifically expressed in different steps of germ cell development should shed new light on the mechanisms of spermatogenesis.

We have cloned germ-cell-specific genes using monoclonal (Watanabe et al. 1994) or polyclonal (Tsuchida et al. 1998; Uchida et al. 2000) antibodies that specifically recognize germ cells at various stages of differentiation. We have also cloned haploid germ-cell-specific cDNAs from a subtracted cDNA library that was generated by subtracting the mRNA of 17-day-old mouse testes (before haploid germ cells develop) from the cDNA of 35-day-old mouse testes (Tanaka et al. 1994; Iguchi et al. 1999). Detailed mRNA expression analysis revealed that the genes corresponding to the cloned cDNAs were exclusively expressed in germ cells at all steps of differentiation, at specific steps of differentiation, or at specific steps in the development of haploid germ cells. The expression of all of these genes was developmentally controlled (Fig. 1).

5.3 Functional Analysis of Gene Products

Male haploid germ cell differentiation, which is also known as spermiogenesis, involves nuclear condensation, the elimination of most of the spermatid cytoplasm, and the formation of the tail and acrosome. During this time period, the cell cycle of haploid spermatids is arrested and

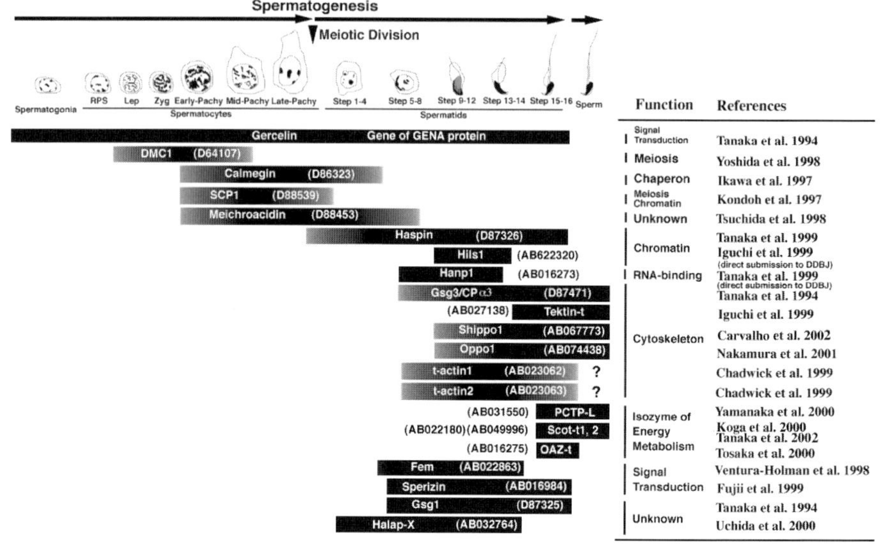

Fig. 1. Germ-cell-specific genes that have been cloned and characterized in our laboratory. The *numbers in parentheses* indicate the DDBJ accession numbers. The *bars* indicate the expression periods of each gene. All of these genes show expression that is developmentally controlled

the transcription of haploid germ-cell-specific genes is stringently regulated. Translation is also regulated by specific molecules that bind RNA and maintain translation in the absence of transcription (Hecht, 1998). During spermiogenesis, RNA-binding proteins may also play an important role in regulating temporal translation by the addition of polyA sequences, or via interactions with *cis*-acting elements in the 5'- and 3'-UTRs of certain genes (Palmiter et al. 1993; Lee et al. 1996; Gu and Hecht, 1996; Braun, 1998). The expression of specific genes appears to be regulated by alternative splicing of their transcripts (Walker et al. 1999; Kleene 2001). Some of the RNA-binding proteins may also play roles in germ-cell-specific mRNA splicing (Moussa et al. 1994; Morales et al. 1997; Elliott et al. 2000). Furthermore, we found novel genes that were involved in mRNA metabolism or chromatin transition in spermiogenesis, and novel DNA-binding proteins, including putative transcription factors, whose precise functions are currently under investigation (Fig. 1).

Germ cell-specific histones and HMG genes (Boissonneault and Lau 1993) might influence chromatin condensation by releasing histones and replacing them with protamines via transition proteins (Baarends et al. 1998). It is generally believed that transcription and translation are repressed during the differentiation process of spermiogenesis. However, the isolation and characterization of haploid germ-cell-specific genes showed that the transcription of specific genes occurred from the highly condensed nucleus, even in very late stages of spermiogenesis. The synthesis of OAZ-t (Fig. 1) and some of the haploid germ-cell-specific cytoskeletal proteins (Fig. 1) are examples of late-transcribed genes. Haploid gene expression also occurs in the case of TBP (TATA-binding protein), and this protein accumulates at much higher levels in early-haploid germ cells than in any other somatic cell type (Schmidt and Schibler 1997). TF IIB and RNA polymerase II are also overexpressed in the testis (Schmidt and Schibler 1995). Furthermore, TPAP (Kashiwabara et al. 2000), EEL3 (Miller et al. 2000) Elongin 2A (Aso et al. 2000), TFIIAtau (Ozer et al. 2000) and TAF (Freiman et al. 2001; Hiller et al. 2001) are specifically expressed in the testis.

Some of the haploid germ-cell-specific genes encoded products that were either involved in energy metabolism or represented germ-cell-specific isozymes of previously known enzymes. These genes were also expressed at specific stages of germ cell differentiation, although the physiological roles of these isozymes remain to be elucidated (Hecht, 1998; Eddy et al. 1998).

The production of large numbers of sperm usually guarantees successful fertilization, and infertility is often related to azoospermia or oligospermia (Jaffe and Oates 1997). However, vertebrate haploid germ cells, unlike those in yeasts and some insects (Ross et al. 1993), do not divide after meiotic division and therefore, rather than proliferating, they differentiate into sperm by complex morphogenesis. Cell-cycle arrest after meiosis commits cells to morphogenetic differentiation during spermiogenesis, and is an important physiological event in a wide range of organisms (Douglas et al. 1998). However, the molecular mechanisms involved in this process are unclear. The *haspin* gene, which encodes a unique nuclear protein kinase, was previously identified in murine testicular haploid germ cells (Tanaka et al. 1999). Ectopic expression of the Haspin protein in cultured somatic cells caused cell-cycle arrest at G1. We speculate that *haspin* plays a role in cell-cycle regulation after meiosis in haploid germ cells.

5.4 Genomic Construction of Haploid Germ-Cell-Specific Genes

We isolated the genomic DNA of haploid-specific genes and identified a number of regulatory motifs in the gene-promoter regions that were essential for transcription. One of these motifs, the cyclic AMP response element, was present in the promoter regions of several testis-specific genes, and was deemed to be functionally important. When the CRE modulator protein (CREM) was deleted using gene targeting in homozygous male mice, spermiogenesis was arrested in the early stages (Nantel et al. 1996). Recently, we cloned the *haspin* (Tanaka et al. 2001a; Yoshimura et al. 2001), *gsg3/Cpα3* (Yoshimura et al. 1999) and *scot-t* genes (Tanaka et al. 2002), all of which show temporal expression during spermiogenesis. Although CRE motifs were found in the 5′-flanking regions of *gsg3/Cpα3* and *scot-t* in both mice and humans, the *haspin* gene-promoter region did not contain a CRE motif. Similarly, the promoter regions of the MMP-28 (Illman et al. 2001), Hormone-sensitive lipase (Blaise et al. 2001), ldhc (Jethanandani and Goldberg 2001), SP-10 (Reddi et al. 1999) genes, which were specifically expressed in haploid germ cells, did not contain CRE motifs. These findings suggest the existence of different haploid germ-cell-specific regulatory proteins that specifically regulate the expression of haploid germ-cell-specific genes.

An interesting feature of the haploid germ-cell-specific genes is that they are intronless. We observed a surprisingly high frequency of intronless genes (41% of the cloned genes). Although some of the functions of intronless genes, in particular those that are specifically expressed in haploid germ cells, have previously been reported (Table 1), our observation of numerous intronless haploid germ-cell-specific genes is novel. Two of the intronless genes, the phosphoglycerate kinase-2 (PGK-2) (McCarrey and Thomas, 1987; McCarrey, 1987) and pyruvate dehydrogenase subunit e2α (PDH) (Dahl et al. 1990) genes, are localized on autosomes, and are believed to be derived by transposon-mediated re-

Table 1. High-frequency expression of intronless genes in the testis

Gene name	Putative original gene	References
PGK-Z	PGK-1	McCarrey and Thomas 1987
Zfα	Zfx	Ashworth et al. 1990
PDHA2	PDHA1	Dahl et al. 1990
MYCL2	MYCL1	Robertson et al. 1991
Protamine3	Protamine1	Schluter and Engel 1995
G6pd2	G6pd1	Hendriksen et al. 1997
Sycpl-ps2	Sycp1	Sage et al. 1997
Pabp2	Pabp1	Kleene et al. 1998
cγ	Cα	Reinton et al. 1998
Cetnl	Cetn2	Hart et al. 1999
Gk-rs1, 2	Gyk	Pan et al. 1999
Gsg3	CPα	Yoshimura et al. 1999
TPAP	PAPII	Lee et al. 2001
Scot-t	Scot	Tanaka et al. 2002
Tsk-1, -2		Galili et al. 1997
SRY		Su and Lau 1993
C15orf2		Farber et al. 2000
Tact1, 2		Chadwick et al. 1999
Haspin		Yoshimura et al. 2001

verse transcription of ancestral genes on the X chromosome. Why do intronless genes translocate to autosomes by retrotransposition? A possible explanation is that translocation provides a means to escape X chromosome inactivation during spermatogenesis (McCarrey and Thomas 1987). The origins of the PGK-2 and PDH genes suggest the involvement of retrotransposons. However, *haspin* (Fig. 2), *gsg3/Cpα3* and *scot-t* (Fig. 3) do not have ancestral counterpart genes on the X chromosome. Alternatively, the intronless genes may have been produced by some other mechanism. In any case, it is likely that specific mechanisms exist in haploid germ-cell-specific genes that conserve an unusually large number of intronless genes. Further detailed studies of other haploid germ cell-specific genes might resolve these issues.

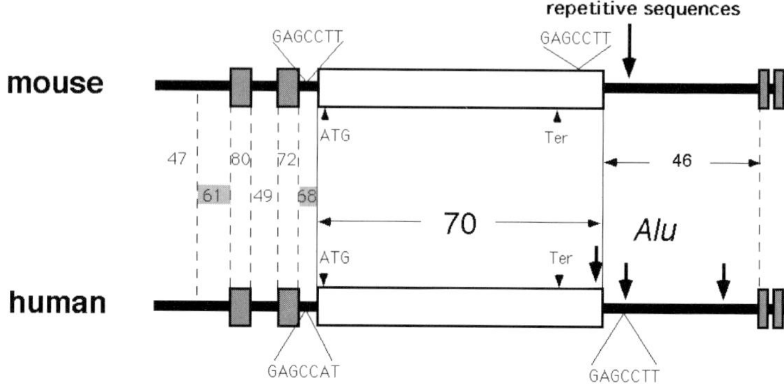

Fig. 2. Schematic representation of the human and mouse *haspin* genes. The intronless *haspin* gene is located in an intron of the integrin alpha E gene. Two genes are transcribed in different directions; the *haspin* mRNA is transcribed starting 49 nucleotides upstream of the ATG translation initiation signal in the rightward direction. The *boxes* indicate the transcribed regions. *Shadowed boxes* indicate exons of the mouse integrin M290 and human integrin alpha E genes. The *numbers* indicate the sequence similarities (%) in each limited region the mouse repetitive and human *Alu* sequences exist in 3′ region (*arrows*). Direct repeats of the GAGCC(T/A)T sequence are located at both ends of the flanking region of the *haspin* gene. The translational start and stop codons are indicated by *ATG* and *Ter*, respectively (*arrowheads*). Sequence of coding regions of both *haspin* and integrin shows more than 70% similarity between mouse and human. The sequence similarity between the flanking regions is less than 50%, except for two 5′-flanking regions that show 61% and 68% similarity (*shadowed numbers*). These regions may be important for developmentally controlled expression of the *haspin* genes in both mice and humans. *Bar*, 1 kb

5.5 Germ Cell Proliferation and Differentiation

Molecular embryology and embryological technology allow us to define the functions of genes that are involved in cell differentiation and normal embryonal development. The introduction of specific genes into early embryos (to create transgenic animals) facilitates studies of gene function and regulation. Although the technique of gene targeting to produce knockout animals allows the study of gene function in vivo, it is both time-consuming and laborious to breed and raise the knockout

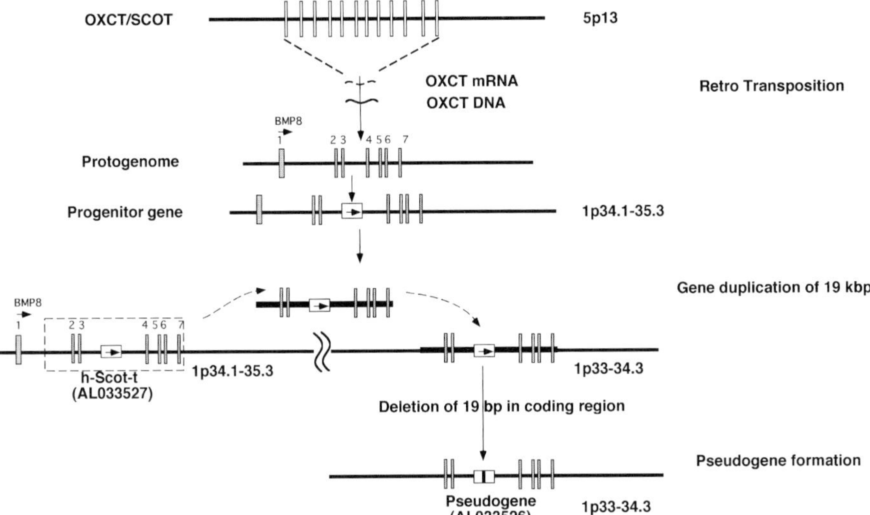

Fig. 3. Schematic representation of the human *Scot-t* gene and flanking region and its evolution. The *open boxes* in OXCT/SCOT show the exons of the somatic-type human *OXCT* gene. The *shadowed boxes* show the exons of the *BMP8* gene. *Open boxes with arrows* show the intronless *scot-t* genes; the *arrows* indicate the direction of transcription for each gene. In theory, the mRNA of *OXCT/SCOT* was retrotransposed to the hypothetical protogenome, and gave rise to an ancestral gene that was subsequently duplicated. One version of the gene was conserved and became the true gene (*left side*), whereas the other gene changed to a pseudogene through deletion and mutation (*right side*) (Tanaka et al., 2001b, 2002)

mice. Recently, a new technique to inject cells and materials into seminiferous tubules has been developed, which makes it possible to study the proliferation and differentiation of ectopic germ cells within the seminiferous tubules of recipient mice (Brinster and Avarbock 1994; Brinster and Zimmermann 1994). In this system, the transplanted cells undergo spermatogenesis and the recipients are capable of transmitting the donor haplotype to the progeny.

We have transplanted the green germ cells of EGFP transgenic mice and measured the proliferation and differentiation of the colonized spermatogonial stem cells in real time (Ohta et al. 2000; Ohta et al.

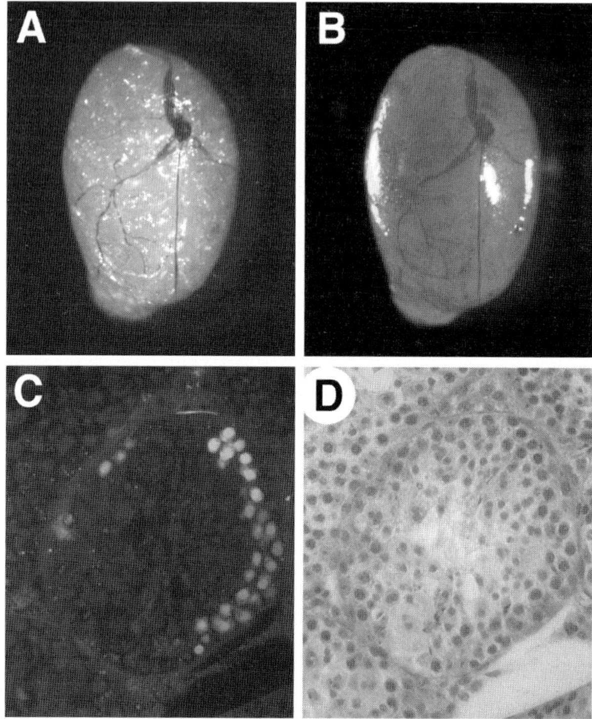

Fig. 4A–D. Transformation and expression of EGFP in seminiferous tubules. After injection of EGFP-cDNA and a blue-dye solution, the whole testis was electrocharged. Two days later, all the blue seminiferous tubules express EGFP which can be traced by fluorescence. Fluorescence can be seen in both germ and Sertoli cells. Low-magnification fluorescence stereomicroscopic views of testes, 2 days after electroporation with the EGFP expression vector (**A**), and the same view under bright-field illumination (**B**). Cross-section of a transfected testis under excitatory light (**C**), and the same section stained with hematoxylin (**D**). The transfected germ cells were detected as positively fluorescing cells

2001). Since efficient in vitro culturing systems have not yet been developed for germ cells, microinjection and cultivation of germ cells in seminiferous tubules is an effective technique for the study of germ cells. By developing methods to transfect germ cells with cDNAs and infect them into seminiferous tubules in vitro, it would be possible to study the roles of gene products from germ cells in their differentiation. The microinjection of cDNA into seminiferous tubules and in vivo electroporation provide useful methods for the efficient transformation of cDNAs into testicular germ cells and Sertoli cells (Yomogida et at, in preparation) (Fig. 4).

5.6 SNP Analysis and Male Infertility

Since almost all mouse male germ-cell-specific genes have human orthologues, the isolation and characterization of counterpart human genes is possible. We expected that mutations in male germ-cell-specific genes in humans would give rise to male infertility. Our strategy was to compare the DNA sequences of fertile and infertile men. Mutations in housekeeping genes would result in loss of function, thereby affecting embryogenesis or somatic cell functions and leading to some defects or illness. In contrast, even if the germ-cell-specific genes were totally defective, the phenotype would be limited to germ cells and the only repercussion would be infertility. Furthermore, since some of the germ-cell-specific genes are intronless, it is easier to examine SNPs or detect mutations by direct DNA sequencing of the PCR products of chromosomal DNA from blood samples (Fig. 5).

Approximately 13% of all couples suffer from infertility, and both female and male factors are known to contribute equally to this disorder (Chandley 1979; Van Assche et al. 1996). Reductions in sperm counts have been reported (Carlsen et al. 1992), although a link with male infertility remains controversial (Sharpe, 1993). Exposure to artificial chemicals is increasingly common, and some of these chemicals may act as endocrine disrupters (ED) to cause defects in spermatogenesis that lead to infertility (U.S. Environmental Protection Agency 1998). To solve these problems, it is important to understand the basic mechanisms of spermatogenesis. Given that a lot of germ-cell-specific genes are not expressed in any other organs or somatic cells, loss-of-function

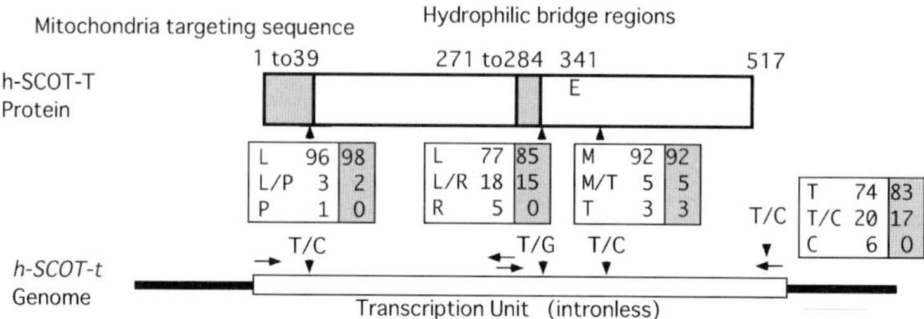

Fig. 5. Schematic representation of SNPs in the haploid germ-cell-specific *scot-t* gene. The transcription unit is represented by an *open box. Arrows* show the primers that were used to avoid the PCR amplification of the pseudogene and to directly sequence SNPs in the human genome. The *shadowed box* in the protein sequence shows the mitochondrial targeting sequence (the N-terminal 39 amino acid residues), and the hydrophilic bridge regions (amino acid residues 271–284). The letter *E* refers to the active-site glutamate (341 amino acid residues) of the SCOT enzyme. *Arrowheads* indicate the sites of a single nucleotide polymorphism and an amino acid variation. The *numbers in the boxes* indicate the percentages of SNPs at each position. The percentages of infertile (270 men in total) and fertile (60 men in total) are shown by *open* and *shadowed boxes*, respectively. Percentages in 3′-UTR are indicated in the *box* by each nucleotide. The *numbers in parentheses* indicate amino acid and nucleotide positions

mutations in these genes (unlike those in housekeeping genes) should lead only to infertility. Therefore, it is important to characterize the molecules that are directly or intimately associated with infertility.

5.7 Future Prospects

Progress in molecular biological techniques adds to our understanding of the regulation of specific molecules that are involved in germ cell differentiation, the relationships between gene products and their physiological roles, and the morphological changes that occur during cell differentiation. The combination of these factors enhances our knowledge and appreciation of spermatogenesis.

References

Aso T, Yamazaki K, Amimoto K, Kuroiwa A, Higashi H, Matsuda Y, Kitajima S, Hatakeyama M (2000) Identification and characterization of Elongin A2, a new member of the Elongin family of transcription elongation factors, specifically expressed in the testis. J Biol Chem 275: 6546-6552

Ashworth A, Skene B, Swift S, Lovell-Badge R (1990) Zfa is an expressed retroposon derived from an alternative transcript of the Zfx gene. EMBO J. 9: 1529–1534

Baarends MW, Roest PH, Hoogerbrugge WJ, Hendriksen MPJ, Hoeijmakers JJH, Grootegoed AJ (1998) Chromatin Structure and gene expression during spermotogenesis. In: M. Stefanini, C. Boitani, M. Galdieri, R. Geremia F. Palomibi (Eds) Testicular Function: From Gene Expression to Genetic Manipulation. Springer-Verlag, Germany, pp 83–103

Bellve AR, O'Brien, DA (1983) The mammalian spermatozoon: structure and temporal assembly. In: Hartmann, JF (ed) Mechanism and Control of Animal Fertilization, Academic Press, New York, USA, pp 55–237.

Blaise R, Guillaudeux T, Tavernier G, Daegelen D, Evrard B, Mairal A, Holm C, Jegou B, Langin D (2001) Testis hormone-sensitive lipase expression in spermatids is governed by a short promoter in transgenic mice. J Biol Chem 276: 5109-51015

Boissonneault G, Lau YF (1993) A testis-specific gene encoding a nuclear high-mobility-group box protein located in elongating spermatids. Mol Cell Biol 13: 4323–4330

Braun RE (1998) Represion and activation of protamine mRNA translation during murine spermatogenesis. In: Zirkin RB (Ed) Germ Cell Development, Division, Disruption and Death. Springer-Verlag, NY, USA, pp 235–251

Brinster RL, Avarbock MR (1994) Germline transmission of donor haplotype following spermatogonial transplantation. Proc Natl Acad Sci USA 91: 11303-11307

Brinster RL, Zimmermann JW (1994) Spermatogenesis following male germ-cell transplantation. Proc Natl Acad Sci USA. 91: 11298-112302

Carlsen E, Giwercman A, Keiding N, Skakkebaek NE (1992) Evidence for decreasing quality of semen during past 50 years. BMJ 305: 609-613

Carvalho EC, Tanaka H, Iguchi N, Ventela S., Nojima H, Nishimune Y (2002) Molecular Cloning and Characterization of a cDNA Encoding Sperm Tail Protein SHIPPO 1. Biol Reprod In press

Chadwick BP, Mull J, Helbling LA, Gill S, Leyne M, Robbins CM, Pinkett HW, Makalowska I, Maayan C, Blumenfeld A, Axelrod FB, Brownstein M, Gusella JF, Slaugenhaupt SA (1999) Cloning, mapping, and expression of two novel actin genes, actin-like-7 A (ACTL7 A) and actin-like-7B

(ACTL7B), from the familialdysautonomia candidate region on 9q31. Genomics 58: 302-309

Chandley AC (1979) The chromosomal basis of human infertility. Br Med Bull 35: 181-186

Clermont Y (1963) The cycle of the seminiferous epithelium cycle in man. Am J Anat 112: 35–51

Dahl HH, Brown RM, Hutchison WM, Maragos C, Brown GK (1990) A testis-specific form of the human pyruvate dehydrogenase E1 alpha subunit is coded for by an intronless gene on chromosome 4. Genomics 8: 225–232

Douglas L, Pittman LD, Schimenti CJ (1998) Recombination and the mammalian germ line. In: Handel AM (ed) Meiosis and Gametogenesis. Academic Press, CA, USA, pp 1–35

Eddy ME and O'Brien, AD (1998) Gene expression during mammalian meiosis. In: Handel AM (Ed) Meiosis and Gametogenesis. Academic Press, CA, USA, pp. 141–200

Elliott DJ, Bourgeois CF, Klink A, Stevenin J, Cooke HJ (2000) A mammalian germ cell-specific RNA-binding protein interacts with ubiquitously expressed proteins involved in splice site selection. Proc Natl Acad Sci USA 97: 5717-5722

Farber C, Gross S, Neesen J, Buiting K, Horsthemke B (2000) Identification of a testis-specific gene (C15orf2) in the Prader-Willi syndrome region on chromosome 15. Genomics 65: 174–183

Freiman RN, Albright SR, Zheng S, Sha WC, Hammer RE, Tjian R (2001) Requirement of tissue-selective TBP-associated factor TAFII105 in ovarian development. Science 293: 2084-2087

Fujii T, Tamura K, Copeland NG, Gilbert DJ, Jenkins NA, Yomogida K, Tanaka H, Nishimune Y, Nojima H, Abiko Y (1999) Sperizin is a murine RING zinc-finger protein specifically expressed in Haploid germ cells. Genomics 57: 94–101

Galili N, Baldwin HS, Lund J, Reeves R, Gong W, Wang Z, Roe BA, Emanuel BS, Nayak S, Michanin C, Budarf ML, Buck CA (1997) A region of mouse chromosome 16 is syntenic to the DiGeorge, velocardiofacial syndrome minimal critical region. Genome Res 7: 17–26

Gu W, Hecht NB (1996) Translational of a testis-specific Cu/Zn superoxide dismutase (SOD-1) mRNA is regulated by a 65-kilodalton protein which bind to its 5′ untranslated region. Mol Cell Biol 16: 4335–4543

Hart PE, Glantz JN, Orth JD, Poynter GM, Salisbury JL (1999) Testis-specific murine centrin, Cetn1: Genomic characterization and evidence for retroposition of a gene encoding a centrosome protein. Genomics 60: 111–120

Hecht, N.B. (1998) Molecular mechanisms of male germ cell differentiation. Bioessays 20: 555-561

Heller CG, Clermont Y (1963) Spermatogenesis in man: an estimate of its duration. Science 140: 184–186

Hendriksen PJM, Hoogerbrugge JW, Baarends WM, de Boer P, Vreeburg JTM, Vos EA, van der Lende T, Grootegoed JA (1997) Testis-specific expression of a functional retroposon encoding glucose-6-phosphate dehydrogenease in the mouse. Genomics 41: 350–359

Hiller MA, Lin TY, Wood C, Fuller MT (2001) Developmental regulation of transcription by a tissue-specific TAF homolog. Genes Dev 15: 1021-1030

Iguchi N, Tanaka H, Fujii T, Tamura K, Kaneko Y, Nojima H, Nishimune Y. (1999) Molecular cloning of haploid germ cell-specific tektin cDNA and analysis of the protein in mouse testis. FEBS Lett 456: 315-321

Ikawa M, Wada I, Kominami K, Watanabe D, Toshimori K, Nishimune Y, Okabe M (1997) The putative chaperone calmegin is required for sperm fertility. Nature 387: 607-611

Illman SA, Keski-Oja J, Lohi J (2001) Promoter characterization of the human and mouse epilysin (MMP-28) genes. Gene 275: 185-194

Jaffe T, Oates DR (1997) Genetic aspects of infertility. In: Lipshultz LI, Howards SS (eds) Infertility in the male. 3rd eds. Mosby-Year Book Inc., Missouri, USA, pp 280–304

Jethanandani P, Goldberg E. (2001) ldhc expression in non-germ cell nuclei is repressed by NF-I binding. J Biol Chem 276: 35414-35421

Kashiwabara S, Zhuang T, Yamagata K, Noguchi J, Fukamizu A, Baba T (2000) Identification of a novel isoform of poly(A) polymerase, TPAP, specifically present in the cytoplasm of spermatogenic cells. Dev Biol 228: 106-115

Kleene KC, Mulligan E, Steiger D, Donohue K, Mastragelo MA (1998) The mouse gene encoding the testis-specific isoform of poly(A) binding protein (Pabp2) is an expressed retroposon: Intimations that gene expression in spermatogenic cells facifitates the creation of new genes. J Mol Evol 47: 275–281

Kleene KC. (2001) A possible meiotic function of the peculiar patterns of gene expression in mammalian spermatogenic cells. Mech Dev 106: 3–23

Koga M, Tanaka H, Yomogida K, Nozaki M, Tsuchida J, Ohta H, Nakamura Y, Masai K, Yoshimura Y, Yamanaka M, Iguchi N, Nojima H, Matsumiya K, Okuyama A, Nishimune Y (2000) Isolation and characterization of a haploid germ cell-specific novel complementary deoxyribonucleic acid; testis-specific homologue ofsuccinyl CoA:3-Oxo acid CoA transferase. Biol Reprod 63: 1601-1609

Kondoh N, Nishina Y, Tsuchida J, Koga M, Tanaka H, Uchida K, Inazawa J, Taketo M, Nozaki M, Nojima H, Matsumiya K, Namiki M, Okuyama A, Nishimune Y (1997) Assignment of synaptonemal complex protein 1

(SCP1) to human chromosome 1p13 by fluorescence in situ hybridization and itsexpression in the testis. Cytogenet Cell Genet 78: 103-104

Lee K, Fajardo MA, Braun RE (1996) A testis cytoplasmic RNA-binding protein that has the properties of a translational repressor. Mol Cell Biol 16: 3023–3034

Lee YJ, Ki m H, Chung JH, Lee Y (2001) Testis-specific expression of an intronless gene encoding a human poly(A) polymerase. Mol Cells 11: 379–385

Lele K, Wolgemuth DJ (1998) The role of transcriptional control during spermatogenesis. J Androl 19: 639-649

McCarrey JR (1987) Nucleotide sequence of the promoter region of a tissue specific human retroposon :comparison with its housekeeping progenitor. Gene 61: 291–298

McCarrey JR, Kelwyn T (1987) Human testis-specific PGK gene lacks introns and possesses characteristics of a processed gene. Nature 326: 501–505

Miller T, Williams K, Johnstone RW, Shilatifard A (2000) Identification, cloning, expression, and biochemical characterization of the testis-specific RNA polymerase II elongation factor ELL3. J Biol Chem 275: 32052-32056

Morales CR, Leyne M, el-Alfy M, Oko R (1997) Molecular cloning and developmental expression of a small ribonuclear protein in the mouse testis. Mol Reprod Dev 46: 459-470

Moussa F, Oko R, Hermo L. (1994) The immunolocalization of small nuclear ribonucleoprotein particles in testicular cells during the cycle of the seminiferous epithelium ofthe adult rat. Cell Tissue Res 278: 363-378

Nakamura Y, Tanaka H, Koga M, Miyagawa Y, Iguchi N, de Carvalho EC, Yomogida K, Nozaki M, Nojima H, Matsumiya K, Okuyama A, Nishimune Y (2001) Molecular Cloning and Characterization of OPPO 1: a Haploid Germ Cell-Specific cDNA Encoding Sperm Tail Protein. Biol Reprod submitted

Nantel F, Monaco L, Foulkes, NS et al. (1996) Spermiogenesis deficiency and germ-cell apoptosis in CREM-mutant mice. Nature 380: 159–162

Oakberg EF (1956) Duration of spermatogenesis in the mouse and timing of stages of the cycle of the seminiferous epithelium. Am J Anat 99: 507–516

Ohta H, Yomogida K, Dohmae K, Nishimune Y (2000) Regulation of proliferation and differentiation in spermatogonial stem cells: the role of c-kit and its ligand SCF. Development 127: 2125-2131

Ohta H, Yomogida K, Tadokoro Y, Tohda A, Dohmae K, Nishimune Y (2001) Defect in germ cells, not in supporting cells, is the cause of male infertility in the jsd mutant mouse: proliferation of spermatogonial stem cells without differentiation. Int J Androl 24: 15–23

Olesen C, Hansen C, Bendsen E, Byskov AG, Schwinger E, Lopez-Pajares I, Jensen PK, Kristoffersson U, Schubert R, Van Assche E, Wahlstroem J,

Lespinasse J, Tommerup N (2001) Identification of human candidate genes for male infertility by digital differential display. Mol Hum Reprod 7: 11–20

Ozer J, Moore PA, Lieberman PM (2000) A testis-specific transcription factor IIA (TFIIAtau) stimulates TATA-binding protein-DNA binding and transcription activation. J Biol Chem 275: 122-128

Palmiter RD, Sandgren EP, Koeller DM, Brinster RL (1993) Distal regulatory elements from the mouse metallothionein locus stimulate gene expression in transgenic mice. Mol Cell Biol 13: 5266–5275

Pan Y, Decker WK, Huq AHHM, Craigen WJ (1999) Retrotransposition of glycerol kinase-related genes from the X chromosome to autosomes: Functional and evolutionary aspects. Genomics 59: 282–290

Reddi PP, Flickinger, CJ, Herr JC (1999) Round spermatid-specific transcription of the mouse SP-10 gene is mediated by a 294-base pair proximal promoter. Biol Reprod 61: 1256-1266

Reinton N, Haugen TB, Orstavik S, Skalhegg BS, Hansson V, Jahnsen T, Tasken K (1998) The gene encoding the C gamma catalysic subunit of cAMP-dependent protein kinase is a transcribed retroposon. Genomics 49: 290–297

Ross, KG, Vargo, EL, Keller L. Trager JC. (1993) Effect of a founder event on variation in the genetic sex-determining system of the fire ant Solenopsis invicta. Genetics 135; 843-854

Robertson NG, Pomponio RJ, Mutter GL, Morton CC (1991) Testis-specific ecxpression of the human MYCL2 gene. Nucleic Acids Res 19: 3129–3137

Russell LD, Ettlin RA, Sinha HAP, Clegg ED (1990) Mammalian Spermatogenesis. In: Russell LD, Ettlin RA, Sinha HAP, Clegg ED (eds) Histological and Histopathological Evaluation of the Testis. Cache River Press, Florida, USA, pp 1–40

Sage J, Yuan L, Martin L, Mattei MG, Guenet JL, Liu JG, Hoog C, Rassoulzadegan M, Cuzin F (1997) The Sycp1 loci of the mouse genome: successive retropositions of a meiotic gene during the recent evolution of the genus. Genomics 44: 118–126

Schluter G, Engel W (1995) The rat Prm3 gene is an intronless member of the protamine gene cluster and is expressed in haploid male germ cells. Cytogenet Cell Genet 71: 352–355

Schmidt EE, Schibler U (1995) High accumulation of components of the RNA polymerase II transcription machinery in rodent spermatids. Development 121: 2373-2383

Schmidt EE, Schibler U (1997) Developmental testis-specific regulation of mRNA levels and mRNA translational efficiencies for TATA-binding protein mRNA isoforms. Dev Biol 184: 138-149

Sharpe RM (1993) Declining sperm counts in men–is there an endocrine cause? J Endocrinol 136: 357-360

Su H, Lau YF (1993) Identification of the transcriptional unit, structural organization, and promoter sequence of the human sex-determining rgion Y (SRY) gene, using a reverse genetic approach. Am J Hum Genet 52: 24–38

Tanaka H, Yoshimura Y, Nishina Y, Nozaki M, Nojima H, Nishimune Y. (1994) Isolation and characterization of cDNA clones specifically expressed in testicular germ cells. FEBS Lett 355: 4–10

Tanaka H, Okabe M, Ikawa M, Tsuchida J, Yoshimura Y, Yomogida K, Nishimune Y. (1998) Studies on the Mechanism of Sperm Production. In: M. Stefanini, C. Boitani, M. Galdieri, R. Geremia F. Palomibi (Eds) Testicular Function: From Gene Expression to Genetic Manipulation. Springer-Verlag, Germany, pp 235–251

Tanaka H, Yoshimura Y, Nozaki M, Yomogida K, Tsuchida J, Tosaka Y, Habu T, Nakanishi T, Okada M, Nojima H, Nishimune Y (1999) Identification and characterization of a haploid germ cell-specific nuclear protein kinase (Haspin) in spermatid nuclei and its effects on somatic cells. J Biol Chem 274: 17049-17057

Tanaka H, Iguchi N, Nakamura Y, Kohroki J, de Carvalho CE, Nishimune Y (2001a) Cloning and characterization of human haspin gene encoding haploid germ cell-specific nuclear protein kinase. Mol Hum Reprod 7: 211-218

Tanaka H, Kohroki J, Iguchi N, Onishi M, Nishimune Y (2002) Cloning and characterization of a human orthologue of testis-specific succinyl CoA: 3-oxo acid CoA transferase (Scot-t) cDNA. Mol Hum Reprod 8:16–23

Tanaka H, Koga M, Iguchi N, Nozaki M, Ohnishi M, Carvalho EC, Nakamura Y, Miyagawa Y, Takeyama M, Matsumiya K, Okuyama A, Nishimune Y (2001b) Andrology in the 21th Centurey: Proceeding of the VIIth International Congress of Andrology. In: Robaire B, Chemes H, Morales RC (Eds) Isolation and characterization of haploid germ cell-specific OXTC cDNAs; Testis-Specific Succinyl CoA: 3-oxo acid CoA transferases (scot-t1 and scot-t2). MEDIMOND, Italy, pp 157–161

Tosaka Y, Tanaka H, Yano Y, Masai K, Nozaki M, Yomogida K, Otani S, Nojima H, Nishimune Y (2000) Identification and characterization of testis specific ornithine decarboxylase antizyme (OAZ-t) gene: expression in haploid germ cells andpolyamine-induced frameshifting. Genes Cells 5: 265-276

Tsuchida J, Nishina Y, Wakabayashi N, Nozaki M, Sakai Y, Nishimune Y. (1998) Molecular cloning and characterization of meichroacidin (male meiotic metaphase chromosome-associated acidic protein). Dev Biol 197: 67–76

Uchida K, Tsuchida J, Tanaka H, Koga M, Nishina Y, Nozaki M, Yoshinaga K, Toshimori K, Matsumiya K, Okuyama A, Nishimune Y. (2000) Cloning and characterization of a complementary deoxyribonucleic acid encoding haploid-specific alanine-rich acidic protein located on chromosome-X. Biol Reprod 63: 993–999

USEPA: Endocrine Disruptor Screening and Testing Advisory Committee (EDSTAC); Final Report (1998) Office of Prevention, Pesticides, and Toxic Substances, U.S. Environmental Protection Agency, Washington DC, USA

Van Assche E, Bonduelle M, Tournaye H, Joris H, Verheyen G, Devroey P, Van Steirteghem A, Liebaers I (1996) Cytogenetics of infertile men. Hum Reprod 11: Suppl 4:1–24; 25-26

Ventura-Holman T, Seldin MF, Li W, Maher JF (1998) The murine fem1 gene family: homologs of the Caenorhabditis elegans sex-determination protein FEM-1. Genomics 54: 221-230

Walker WH, Delfino FJ, Habener JF (1999) RNA processing and the control of spermatogenesis. Front Horm Res 25: 34–58

Watanabe D, Yamada K, Nishina Y, Tajima Y, Koshimizu U, Nagata A, Nishimune Y. (1994) Molecular cloning of a novel Ca(2+)-binding protein (calmegin) specifically expressed during male meiotic germ cell development. J Biol Chem 269: 7744-7749

Yamanaka M, Koga M, Tanaka H, Nakamura Y, Ohta H, Yomogida K, Tsuchida J, Iguchi N, Nojima H, Nozaki M, Matsumiya K, Okuyama A, Toshimori K, Nishimune Y (2000) Molecular cloning and characterization of phosphatidylcholine transfer protein-like protein gene expressed in murine haploid germ cells. Biol Reprod 62: 1694–1701

Yoshida K, Kondoh G, Matsuda Y, Habu T, Nishimune Y, Morita T (1998) The mouse RecA-like gene Dmc1 is required for homologous chromosome synapsis during meiosis. Mol Cell 1: 707-718

Yoshimura Y, Tanaka H, Nozaki M, Yomogida K, Shimamura K, Yasunaga T, Nishimune Y (1999) Genomic analysis of male germ cell-specific actin capping protein alpha. Gene 237: 193-199

Yoshimura Y, Tanaka H, Nozaki M, Yomogida K, Yasunaga T, Nishimune Y (2001) Nested genomic structure of haploid germ cell specific haspin gene. Gene 267: 49–54

6 Control of Spermatogenesis via Sertoli Cells

M.D. Griswold, D. McLean

Every new breakthrough in technology and every new piece of published data reinforces the impression that spermatogenesis is an enormously complex process. This complexity results from the multiple interactions between somatic cells, germinal cells and endocrine signals. Interruptions in many of these interactions can lead to a blockage or impedance of the developmental pathway. As with any complex system, some essential elements of spermatogenesis could be considered "control points" for the entire process. These "control points" are of interest to scientists investigating both infertility and approaches to contraception. Many potential "control points" are represented by individual genes and have come to our attention because of natural or induced mutations that result in aberrant or absent spermatogenesis. A summary of genes whose expression appears to be essential for normal spermatogenesis is available on a web site supported by the National Institute of Child Health and Human Development (NICHD) (see http://www.mouse.genetics.

washington.edu/). This website is maintained by Dr. Robert Braun of the University of Washington and will eventually contain databases of all existing mutants, gene expression patterns and regulatory information, gene array data, links to the primary literature, and a protein linkage map of the spermatozoon.

Many of the genes that are currently known to affect spermatogenesis are expressed in the developing germ cells [1, 2]. There are a number of genes whose expression is essential for meiosis, normal germ cell phenotype, and normal germ cell numbers. In addition, many genes essential for correct endocrine signaling have been identified. Genes that code for GnRH, the gonadotropins, androgen biosynthesis, and the requisite receptors for these signals are clearly key "control points" for spermatogenesis (for a review see [3]). Knowledge of genes that are required for the functions of the somatic cells (Sertoli and peritubular) of the seminiferous tubules is more limited. The determination of exactly which properties or functions of Sertoli cells are crucial in spermatogenesis has been a major research goal in many laboratories.

6.1 Evidence for the Essential Nature of Sertoli Cells

Germinal cells and Sertoli cells have obligatory interactions that begin during testis development and continue in spermatogenesis [3]. When the embryonic testis is formed, Sertoli cells sequester the germ cells (gonocytes) inside of seminiferous tubules and inhibit the penchant of these cells to enter into meiosis. Unsequestered gonocytes in the male or those destined for the ovary in the female enter into meiotic prophase shortly after organ formation [4]. This process of testis formation requires the expression of specific genes on the Y-chromosome. Following testis formation Sertoli cells and germ cells undergo rapid proliferation. The onset of puberty generally involves the cessation of mitosis of Sertoli cells, the formation of tight junctions between adjacent Sertoli cells and the progression of germ cells through meiosis and their differentiation into spermatozoa.

The view that Sertoli cells are essential in spermatogenesis is a result of several observations. First, there is no reported occurrence of testes that contain germ cells but no Sertoli cells. In addition, the ability of germ cells in cell culture to survive and develop independent of co-culture with somatic cells is very limited. Mammalian spermatogenesis cannot be easily demonstrated in culture but when claims for success have been published there is usually a requirement for Sertoli cells. In the amphibian, germinal cells will develop in culture and some elements of this development are independent of the presence of Sertoli cells [5]. However, the advancement of amphibian spermatocytes through meiosis and some aspects of the maturation of spermatids require the presence of Sertoli cells in the co-culture. A similar reliance on Sertoli cells in the mammalian testis can be postulated.

The second observation demonstrating the essential nature of Sertoli cells leads to the conclusion that they are limiting to germ cell numbers. The maximum number of germ cells supported by Sertoli cells varies between species, however, it is constant within a species. This limiting nature of Sertoli cells was demonstrated experimentally when the size of the testis and the spermatogenic output was manipulated by changing the number of Sertoli cells. Orth et al. (1988) inhibited the proliferation of rat Sertoli cells during testicular development which resulted in male offspring with smaller than normal testes [6]. In the converse experiment, propylthiouracil was used to inhibit thyroid hormone action during development and this treatment resulted in rats with larger than normal testes [7]. Hemicastration of developing testes in several mammalian species at the appropriate age results in an increased proliferation of Sertoli cells in the remaining testis with concomitant increase in testicular size. In each of these animal models, the ratio of spermatids to Sertoli cells was relatively constant before and after the treatments. The conclusion is that the number of germ cells appears to be directly related to the number of functional Sertoli cells.

Finally, a third group of experimental observations has led to the conclusion that the endocrine requirement for spermatogenesis in higher vertebrates is a result of the action of reproductive hormones such as FSH and testosterone on Sertoli cells and not on germ cells.

6.2 FSH and Testosterone Control Spermatogenesis via Sertoli Cells

The availability of antibodies to the androgen receptors has led to the demonstration of receptors in Sertoli and peritubular cells (for a review see [13]). Evidence for the lack of androgen action directly on germ cells in the testis was originally obtained from genetic studies [14]. More recently, the spermatogonial stem cell transplantation technique was employed to determine if murine germ cells require functional androgen receptors to complete qualitatively normal spermatogenesis [15]. The gene for the androgen receptor is found on the X-chromosome and in mice bearing the testicular feminization mutation (*Tfm*) where functional androgen receptors are absent, a testis is formed and germ cell development proceeds only as far as primary spermatocytes. Germ cells from testicular feminized mice were injected into the seminiferous tubules of azoospermic mice expressing functional androgen receptors. Recipient testes were analyzed between 110 and 200 days following transplantation and multiple colonies of complete and qualitatively normal donor-derived spermatogenesis were seen within the seminiferous tubules of each recipient testis. This result clearly demonstrated that murine germ cells do not require functional androgen receptors to complete spermatogenesis.

Androgen action on Sertoli cells and peritubular cells is essential for spermatogenesis and despite detailed molecular information on the androgen receptor, there is little reliable information about the molecular events stimulated by testosterone [16]. The molecular mode of action of testosterone in spermatogenesis remains a major puzzle.

The role of FSH in spermatogenesis has been controversial [17]. Some recent experiments have helped to clarify the overall biological role of FSH. Handelsman and colleagues administered testosterone alone to gonadotropin releasing hormone (GnRH) deficient mice and showed that this treatment alone led to testicular maturation and fertility [18]. GnRH deficient mutant mice treated with testosterone implants had normal spermatogenesis but reduced testis size and germ cell numbers. In a parallel study the same group showed that FSH treatment, in addition to testosterone treatment, resulted in GnRH deficient mice with quantitatively normal spermatogenesis and testes of normal size [19]. The authors concluded from these studies that FSH treatment during the first 2 weeks of life increased Sertoli cell numbers and total sperm production in the mouse testis. It has also been demonstrated that prepubertal treatment of normal rats with additional FSH produced larger than normal testes and higher numbers of germ cells [20]. In other experiments, a FSH β gene knock-out has resulted in a line of mice where the males were fertile but had smaller than normal testes and reduced numbers of germ cells [21]. A FSH receptor null mutation (566C->T) has been reported in 5 male humans [22]. The men showed variable degrees of spermatogenic failure but were not infertile. None of the 5 men had normal sperm parameters and testicular size was reduced but two of the men had fathered two children each. These results in summary clearly showed that FSH is not required for fertility in mice or men but there is a role for FSH in testis size and ultimately in numbers of sperm produced.

6.3 Requirement for Sertoli Cells in Spermatogenesis

Sertoli cells provide critical features necessary for successful spermatogenesis. These critical features may include the physical support of germ cells, the formation of junctional complexes or barriers, or biochemical stimulation in the form of growth factors and nutrients (Table 1). There are a number of excellent reviews dealing with this topic [23–31]. There is experimental evidence that the breakdown of the tight junctional complexes and two compartment system in the testis quickly leads to aspermatogenesis. The biochemical products of Sertoli cells form a unique and essential environment for germ cell spermatogenesis in the adluminal compartment. Some of the products of Sertoli cells may not be absolute requirements for spermatogenesis but may influence the efficiency of the process.

Sertoli cells make and secrete a number of proteins that form the molecular basis for the Sertoli-germ cell interactions [25, 32, 33]. The glycoproteins secreted by the Sertoli cells can be placed in several categories based on their known biochemical properties (Table 1). In addition to these proteins, Sertoli cells may secrete bioactive peptides such as prodynorphin and nutrients or metabolic intermediates.

The proposed function for the glycoproteins in the process of spermatogenesis is inferred from the known properties of the proteins. One

Table 1. Types of proteins secreted by Sertoli cells

Category	Proposed function or examples
Transport or bioprotective	Metal ion transport such as transferrin, small molecule transport
Proteases and inhibitors	Tissue remodeling, spermiation
Basement membrane proteins	Formation of a portion of the basement membrane
Regulatory glycoproteins	Müllerian inhibiting substance (MIS), *c kit* ligand, and inhibin

of the most completely described function for a product of Sertoli cells is the role of transferrin which is an iron transport protein also made in the liver and the brain. Sertoli cells make transferrin as part of a proposed iron shuttle system that effectively transports iron around the tight junction complexes to the developing germ cells [34]. The proposed model includes basal transferrin receptors on Sertoli cells, movement of iron through the cell, secretion of ferric ions associated with a newly synthesized testicular transferrins and incorporation of iron in the newly synthesized transferrin into ferritin in the developing germ cells. Most aspects of this model have been experimentally verified in vivo.

6.4 The Transcriptome of Sertoli Cells

Technologies developed because of genome sequencing projects make it possible to ultimately define all of the genes expressed in Sertoli cells. Many Sertoli cell products that have been described in the literature are not unique to Sertoli cells. For example, transferrin is a major Sertoli cell product but also is made in several other tissues including the liver and brain. Of particular interest to understanding the control of spermatogenesis by Sertoli cells are those genes such as the FSH receptor whose expression is limited to Sertoli cells. We have utilized two techniques, PCR differential display and Affymetrix GeneChip arrays to attempt to define those genes whose expression is unique to Sertoli cells. The advantage of the display technology is that unique genes that have not been previously described can be characterized. However, this characterization can be very labor intensive. The advantage of the array

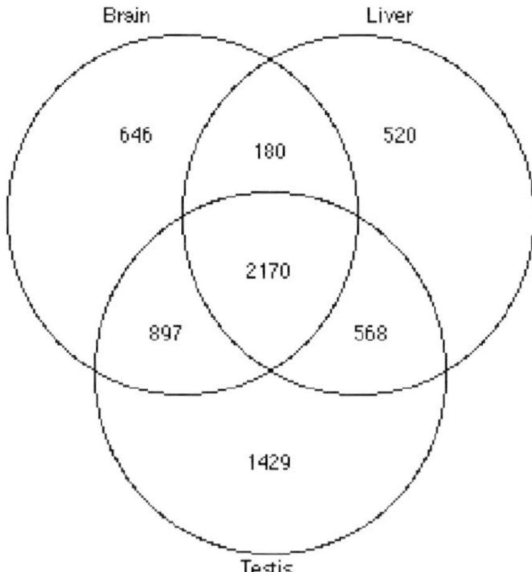

Fig. 1. Venn diagram of the gene expression pattern obtained from U74A GeneChip (12,000 genes) of adult mouse liver, brain and testis. Data were obtained from a single analysis of total RNA isolated in the three tissue types. *Numbers* represent the number of genes present in each cell type (*outer portion of each circle*), the number of gene present in two cell types (*merged portion of two circles*) or the number of genes expressed in all three cell types (*inner portion of all three circles*). Gene presence was determined by absolute analysis on Microarray Suite software. Venn diagram generated by Genespring

technology is that information can be obtained on the expression of thousands of genes in a single experiment. However, this approach requires prior knowledge of the sequence of the expressed gene. The Affymetrix GeneChip system has chips with arrayed oligonucleotides representing thousands of known genes, and the capability to accurately quantify the levels of expressed sequences. The disadvantage of the Affymetrix GeneChip system is that it lacks complete coverage of expressed murine genes at this time although, 36,000 expressed murine sequences are arrayed on 3 GeneChips.

Using the display technique we have described a unique retrovirus related sequence that is specifically expressed in rat Sertoli cells [35]. The promoter for this gene appeared to be active only in Sertoli cells in transfection assays. In addition, we have found two genes from the cystatin family, cystatin SC and cystatin TE-1, that are expressed only in Sertoli cells (SC) or in Sertoli cells and the epididymis (TE-1) [36]. Using the Affymetrix GeneChip system, we are attempting to more broadly define the Sertoli cell transcriptome. In preliminary experiments when we used the GeneChips that contained 12,000 known expressed mouse sequences we found that about 37% of the genes on the chip were expressed in mouse testes. When compared to genes expressed in the mouse brain and liver, 1,420 genes or about 12% were specific to the testis. These data are summarized in Fig. 1, using a Venn diagram. Of the unique testis genes, 492 or about 4% of the genes on the chip were expressed in cultured Sertoli cells. These data underline the complex nature of spermatogenesis and suggests hundreds of potential cell specific gene products expressed exclusively in Sertoli cells are potential regulators of spermatogenesis. The determination of the function of these unique gene products should lead to a deeper understanding of the role of Sertoli cells in controlling spermatogenesis.

References

1. Eddy E.M., D.A.. OB (1998) Gene expression during mammalian meiosis. Curr Top Dev Biol 37:141–200
2. Hecht N (1992) Gene Expression During Male Germ Cell Development. In: Desjardins C, Ewing L (eds) Cell and Molecular Biology of the Testis. Oxford Press, Oxford, Eng., vol 464
3. Griswold MD (1998) The central role of Sertoli cells in spermatogenesis. Semin Cell Dev Biol 9:411–6
4. McLaren A (1984) Meiosis and differentiation of mouse germ cells. Symp Soc Exp Biol 38:7–23
5. Li LY, Seddon AP, Meister A, Risley MS (1989) Spermatogenic cell-somatic cell interactions are required for maintenance of spermatogenic cell glutathione. Biol Reprod 40:317–31
6. Orth JM, Gunsalus GL, Lamperti AA (1988) Evidence from Sertoli cell-depleted rats indicates that spermatid number in adults depends on numbers of Sertoli cells produced during perinatal development. Endocrinology 122:787–94
7. Hess RA, Cooke PS, Bunick D, Kirby JD (1993) Adult testicular enlargement induced by neonatal hypothyroidism is accompanied by increased Sertoli and germ cell numbers. Endocrinology 132:2607–2613

8. Cunningham GR, Tindall DJ, Huckins C, Means AR (1978) Mechanisms for the testicular hypertrophy which follows hemicastration. Endocrinology 102:16–23

9. Kosco MS, Loseth KJ, Crabo BG (1989) Development of the seminiferous tubules after neonatal hemicastration in the boar. J Reprod Fertil 87:1–11

10. Orth JM, Higginbotham CA, Salisbury RL (1984) Hemicastration causes and testosterone prevents enhanced uptake of [3H] thymidine by Sertoli cells in testes of immature rats. Biol Reprod 30:263–70

11. Putra DK, Blackshaw AW (1982) Morphometric studies of compensatory testicular hypertrophy in the rat after hemicastration. Aust J Biol Sci 35:287–93

12. Simorangkir DR, de Kretser DM, Wreford NG (1995) Increased numbers of Sertoli and germ cells in adult rat testes induced by synergistic action of transient neonatal hypothyroidism and neonatal hemicastration. J Reprod Fertil 104:207–13

13. Sar M, Hall SH, Wilson EM, French FS (1993) Androgen Regulation of Sertoli Cells. In: Griswold MD, Russell LD (eds) The Sertoli Cell. Cache River Press, Clearwater, Fl:509–516

14. Fritz I (1978) Sites of actions of androgens and follicle stimulating hormone on cells of the seminiferous tubule. In: Litwack G (ed) Biochemical Actions of Hormones. Academic Press., New York, vol V:249–278.

15. Johnston DS, Russell LD, Friel PJ, Griswold MD (2001) Murine germ cells do not require functional androgen receptors to complete spermatogenesis following spermatogonial stem cell transplantation. Endocrinology 142:2405–2408

16. Tribely W, Roberts K, Griswold MD (1996) Androgen regulation of Sertoli cell function. In: Basin S, Gabelnick S, Spieler J, Swerdloff R, Wang C, Kelley C (eds) Pharmacology, Biology, and Clinical Applications of Androgens. Wily-Liss, New York:11–16

17. Zirken B, Awoniyi, C., Griswold, M., Russel, L., and Sharpe, R. (1994) Is FSH required for Adult Spermatogenesis? J Androl 15:273–276

18. Singh J, O'Neill C, Handelsman DJ (1995) Induction of spermatogenesis by androgens in gonadotropin-deficient (*hpg*) mice. Endocrinology 136:5311–5321

19. Singh J, Handelsman DJ (1996) Neonatal administration of FSH increases Sertoli cell numbers and spermatogenesis in gonadotropin-deficient (*hpg*) mice. J. Endocrinology 151:37–48

20. Meachem SJ, McLachlan R, de Kretser D, Robertson DM, Wreford NG (1996) Neonatal exposure of rats to recombinant follicle stimulating hormone increases adult Sertoli cell and spermatogenic cell numbers. Biol Reprod 54:36–44

21. Kumar TR, Wang Y, Lu N, Matzuk M (1997) Follicle stimulating hormone is required for ovarian follicle maturation but not male fertility. Nat Gen 15:201–204
22. Tapanainen JS, Aittomaki K, Vaskivuo T, Huhtaniemi IT (1997) Men homozygous for an activating mutation of the follicle-stimulating hormone (FSH) receptor gene present variable suppression of spermatogenesis and fertility. Nat Genet 15:205–206
23. Enders G (1993) Sertoli-Sertoli and Sertoli-germ Cell Communications. In: Griswold MD, Russell LD (eds) Ther Sertoli Cell. Cache River Press, Clearwater, FL
24. Fritz IB (1994) Somatic cell-germ cell relationships in mammalian testes during development and spermatogenesis. Ciba Found Symp 182:271–4; discussion 274–81
25. Griswold MD (1995) Interactions between germ cells and Sertoli cells in the testis. Biol Reprod 52:211–6
26. Jegou B (1993) The Sertoli-germ cell communication network in mammals. Int Rev Cytol 147:25–96
27. Kierszenbaum AL (1994) Mammalian Spermatogenesis in Vivo and in Vitro: A Partnership of Spermatogenic and Somatic Cell Lineages. Endocrine Rev 15:116–134
28. McGuinness MP, Griswold MD (1993) Interactions between Sertoli cells and germ cells in the testis. Sem Dev Biol. Submitted
29. Russell LD, Griswold MD (1993) Morphological and Functional Evidence for Sertoli-germ Cell Relationships. In: Griswold MD, Russell LD (eds) Ther Sertoli Cell. Cache River Press, Clearwater, FL
30. Skinner MK (1991) Cell-cell interactions in the testis. Endocr Rev 12:45–77
31. Skinner MK (1993) Sertoli cell-peritubular myoid cell interactions. In: Griswold MD, Russell L (eds) The Sertoli Cell. Cache River Press, Clearwater, FL:477–484
32. Griswold MD (1988) Protein secretions of Sertoli cells. Int Rev Cytol 133–141
33. Griswold MD (1993) Protein secretion by Sertoli cells: general considerations. In: Griswold MD, Russell LD (eds) The Sertoli Cell. Cache River Press, Clarwater, FL:195–200
34. Sylvester SR, Griswold MD (1994) The testicular iron shuttle: a nurse function of the Sertoli cells. J Androl 15:381–5
35. Anway MD, Johnston DS, Crawford D, Griswold MD (2001) A novel retrovirus is expressed specifically in rat Sertoli cells and Granulosa cells. Biol Reprod. 65:1289–1296
36. Li Y, Griswold MD. Submitted

7 Gene-Modified Animal Models for the Study of Luteinizing Hormone and Luteinizing Hormone Receptor Function

F.-P. Zhang, M. Poutanen, I. Huhtaniemi

7.1 Background

Luteinizing hormone (LH), synthesized and secreted by the anterior pituitary gland, and human chorionic gonadotropin (hCG) of placental origin belong together with FSH and thyroid-stimulating hormone (TSH) to the family of glycoprotein hormones. They all are heterodimers composed of two noncovalently associated subunits, the common α-subunit and the hormone-specific β-subunit. The α-subunit is identical in all glycoprotein hormones, whereas different β-subunits determine the hormonal specificity of each glycoprotein hormone. The β-subunits of LH and hCG form an exception: although they are not identical, they are structurally close enough to allow the LH and hCG α/β dimers to bind to the same LH receptor (Gharib et al. 1990). All glycoprotein hormone receptors belong to a subgroup of G-protein-coupled receptors with a unique large extracellular domain. LHR consists of

11 exons [10 exons in the monkey (Zhang et al. 1997)], and the first 10 of them (9 in monkey) encode for the extracellular domain. The last long exon 11 (10 in monkey) encodes a part of the extracellular domain as well as the transmembrane and cytoplasmic domains, which are coupled to the LH signal transduction system (Segaloff and Ascoli 1993; Tena-Sempere and Huhtaniemi 1999).

LHR is mainly expressed in Leydig cell in the testis, and in theca, stromal, late-stage granulosa and luteal cells in the ovary. Upon LH binding to its receptor, Leydig cell androgen production is stimulated, an effect indispensable for maintenance of the endocrine (extratesticular) and paracrine (spermatogenic) effects of androgens (Segaloff and Ascoli 1993; Saez 1994). In the ovary, LH stimulates androgen production of theca cells, thus providing substrate for granulosa cell estrogen production. In addition, it triggers ovulation and maintains the progesterone production of corpus luteum (Richards 1994, 2001; Richards et al. 1995). The synthesis and secretion of LH are under positive control of the hypothalamic gonadotropin-releasing hormone (GnRH), and gonadal steroid and peptide hormones exert negative and positive feedback effects on gonadotropin synthesis and secretion, either directly at the pituitary level or indirectly via the hypothalamus, mainly by modulating GnRH secretion.

A considerable body of novel information on the function of LH and its receptor has been obtained recently through unraveling of phenotypes of activating and inactivating human mutations of the LHR gene (for a review, see Themmen and Huhtaniemi 2000). Activating LHR mutations result in familial male-limited precocious puberty ("testotoxicosis"), but no phenotype has been identified in females. Depending on completeness of the LHR inactivation, the numerous men detected present with phenotypes ranging from micropenis and hypospadias to complete sex reversal, i.e. pseudohermaphroditism. The consequences of inactivation of LH function are still incompletely known, because only a single man with LHβ mutation has so far been reported (Weiss et al. 1992), and no animal model for LHβ knockout (KO) exists yet. The male with LHβ inactivation presented with normal sexual differentiation at birth but total lack of postnatal sexual development. No women with such mutation have yet been found. The animal models for targeted disruption of the gonadotropin subunit and receptor genes (Kendall et al. 1995; Kumar et al. 1997; Dierich et al. 1998; Abel et al. 2000; Lei et al.

2001; Zhang et al. 2001) have been of great importance, and provided new vistas into functions of these hormones.

7.2 *hpg* Mice

A classical, naturally occurring KO of gonadotropin secretion is the hypogonadotropin *hpg* mice (Cattanach et al. 1977), due to a long deletion in the GnRH gene (Mason et al. 1986a,b). GnRH synthesis and secretion are totally abolished in these mice, and there is consequently a near-total deficiency of both gonadotropins (Charlton 1984). The *hpg* male mice can easily be distinguished in adult age from their normal littermates by external examination: the penis is smaller than normal, the scrotum is underdeveloped, and the anogenital distance is much shorter than in normal males. Internally, all male reproductive organs are present but immature. The testes are very small and located in the abdomen. Testicular histology in adult age shows that spermatogenesis in the majority of seminiferous tubules is hardly advanced beyond the diplotene stage. Testicular interstitial tissue is scanty and appears meta-bolically inactive, in keeping with the key role of gonadotropins in the stimulation of steroidogenesis. The ovary and uterus are rather small in female *hpg* mice. The ovaries contain mainly undeveloped follicles up to the preantral stage, with only a few showing early stages of antrum formation. No luteal tissue is present in the ovary and the interstitial tissue is atrophic.

This mutant mouse has been extensively used as a model to study the phenotypic expression of hypogonadotropic hypogonadism and for its experimental treatments (Charlton 1984). The disadvantage of this model is that the mice with deletion of the GnRH gene still have low levels of gonadotropins, potentially with some residual biological activity (O'Shaughnessy et al. 1998).

7.3 Glycoprotein Hormone Common α-Subunit KO Mice

The glycoprotein hormones, LH, FSH and TSH, are critical for gonadal and thyroid development and function, respectively. They all are com-posed of a common α-subunit and unique β-subunit, and the heterodimerization is required for all of their biological functions. To elucidate the exact developmental roles of the free α-subunit and the dimeric forms of LH, FSH and TSH in vivo, mice with disrupted α-subunit gene were produced by the group of Camper (Kendall et al. 1995).

The targeting construct for α-subunit inactivation was constructed containing the neomycin resistance gene within the third exon of the common α-subunit gene, to disrupt the normal open reading frame (Kendall et al. 1995). In the (-/-) mice, displaying total absence of bioactive LH, FSH and TSH, complete sexual differentiation and fetal genital development occurred normally, as monitored at birth. In males, the epididymides and vasa deferentia were present, providing evidence for complete male sexual differentiation; the differentiation of these structures from the Wolffian duct is known to be testosterone dependent (Desjardins 1981). The presence of epididymis and vas deferences indicates that the (-/-) mice were capable of producing sufficient levels of testosterone during the fetal development. Histological examination of 8-week-old mice revealed smaller semineferous tubules, scant interstitial cells and spermatogenesis arrested at the first meiotic division. The structure of the seminiferous tubules at the age of 8 weeks suggested that they did not develop significantly after birth. Testes of neonatal (-/-) animals presented with tubules exactly at the same developmental stage as in age-matched wild-type (WT) testes, indicating normal testicular development in utero in the absence of gonadotropins. Testosterone production by the Leydig cells is stimulated by pituitary LH in adult animals. There is a growing body of evidence suggesting that fetal testosterone production requires little if any LH stimulation in rodents. For example, the *hpg* mice with inactivated GnRH gene have very low gonadotropin levels despite complete sexual differentiation (Cattanach et al. 1977). However, the possibility remains with this model that the low residual levels of LH could stimulate testosterone production to some extent (O'Shaughnessy et al. 1998). The data on the α-subunit KO mice strengthen the contention that sufficient fetal testicular testosterone production to induce masculinization is possible in rodents in the absence of gonadotropins.

An inactivating mutation of the human LHβ-subunit gene results in a phenotype similar to that found in the α-subunit KO in mice. The single affected male so far detected was infertile, but developed normal male external genitalia in utero, as well as Wolffian duct derivatives (Weiss et al. 1992). Because this inactivating human LHβ-subunit mutation was apparently complete, the different phenotypes detected in humans in connection with the LHR and cognate ligand mutations could mean that the receptor could be partially active in the absence of ligand. Alternatively, and more likely, another ligand such as hCG may stimulate fetal testicular LHR in utero to promote masculinization of the genital structures (Huhtaniemi et al. 1977).

Sexual differentiation is normal also in the common α-subunit (-/-) female mice, but postnatally their ovaries are very small, and the uteri are thread-like and less developed than in age-matched WT mice, indicating lack of sufficient estrogen production (Kendall et al. 1995). Follicles at the age of 8 weeks displayed considerable development in the (-/-) mice, but they remained small and failed to progress to the antral stage or to proceed to ovulation. At birth, the ovaries of (-/-) and (+/+) animals were indistinguishable. Furthermore, ovarian development in the (-/-) animals continued postnatally, but it was arrested around postnatal day 21 which is the age of appearance of antral follicles in WT mice. The data on the (-/-) mice confirmed that the prenatal ovarian development is independent of gonadotropin stimulation. Remarkably, the ovarian follicular development during the infantile period is also gonadotropin independent, shown by the fact that at birth the α-subunit deficient mice have follicles developed to the preantral stage. However, the development of follicles to the antral stage and beyond is dependent on gonadotropins and estrogen. As expected, the extent of follicular development in the common α-subunit KO mice is similar to that observed in *hpg* mice.

7.4 LH Receptor KO (LuRKO) Mice

The naturally occurring KO model, *hpg* mouse, as well as common α-subunit KO mouse, provide useful information regarding the role of gonadotropins in the reproductive functions. However, many details about the exact functions of the two gonadotropins are still unclear. Therefore, we found it important to generate a KO mouse model for disrupted LHR gene function, in addition to the already existing FSHR KO mice (Dierich et al. 1998; Abel et al. 2000).

We targeted the LHR gene in embryonic stem (ES) cells using conventional KO techniques, by replacing exon 11 of the gene with a neomycin cassette (Zhang et al. 2001). After electroporation of the targeting construct into ES cells and drug selection, 250 surviving clones were picked, screened by PCR, and positive clones confirmed by Southern hybridization. Five of the 250 clones demonstrated occurrence of homologous recombination. Three of these cell lines were injected into blastocysts, yielding nine male chimeras. The chimeric males were bread with WT C57BL/6 female mice, and three of them went into the germline. Both male and female heterozygous mice were fertile and viable, and were used to generate homozygous LuRKO mice. Another LHR KO model, with targeted disruption of exon 1 of the LHR gene, was reported simultaneously with our study (Lei et al. 2001).

The male LuRKO and WT mice were indistinguishable at birth, and their testes were similar in size and microscopic appearance (Fig. 1). This demonstrated that the intrauterine process of masculinization, although critically dependent on fetal testicular production of two hormones, testosterone and the anti-Müllerian hormone (AMH), is not dependent on LHR function in the testis. As expected, also the neonatal LuRKO and WT females were indistinguishable, in accordance with the previous knowledge that female sexual differentiation is independent of gonadal function. The finding on males provides direct evidence for a phenomenon already shown earlier by less specific approaches, that the rodent fetal testes are able to produce sufficient amounts of testosterone for male-type differentiation in the absence of gonadotropic stimulation. In support to this, previous studies had shown that the GnRH and gonadotropin deficient *hpg* mice are normally masculinized at birth (Cattanach et al. 1977; O'Shaughnessy et al. 1998). Likewise, KO mice for the glycoprotein hormone common α-subunit gene, devoid of LH, FSH and TSH, are normally masculinized at the time of birth (Kendall et al. 1995), after which their sexual maturation stops completely. Moreover, we have recently found that mice deficient of the *T/ebp* transcription factor, and totally missing differentiation of the pituitary gland, also masculinize normally before birth (P. Pakarinen, S. Kimura, F. El-Gehani, L.J. Pelliniemi, and I. Huhtaniemi, submitted for publication). Hence, evidence is now mounting that fetal pituitary LH production, and LHR stimulation of Leydig cell steroidogenesis, are not necessary for masculinization of fetal male mice.

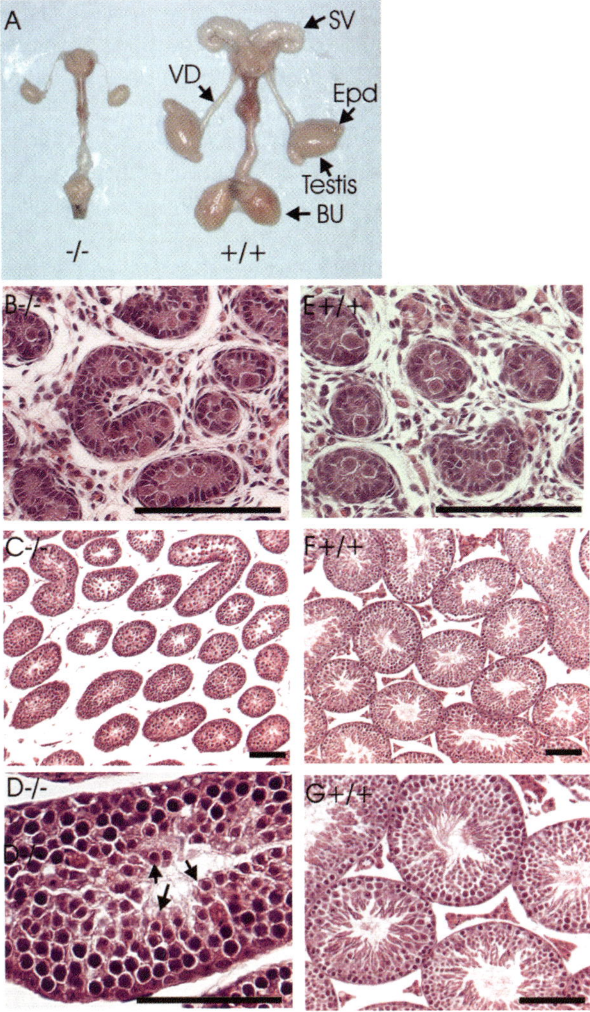

Fig. 1A–G. Morphology and histology of the testes of control WT and homozygous LuRKO male mice. **A** Testes and accessory sex organs of a KO and a WT littermate. *VD*, Vas deferens; *SV*, seminal vesicle; *Epd*, epididymis; *BU*, bulbo-urethral gland. **B**, **E** Testicular histology of a 1-day-old KO and WT mouse. **C**, **F** Testicular histology of a 45-day-old KO and WT mouse. **D**, **G** As in **C** and **F**, at higher magnification. *RS*, round spermatid. *Bar* in panels **B–G**, 100 µm

Although fetal testicular testosterone synthesis is crucial for male sexual differentiation, the LuRKO mice provide, for the first time, direct evidence that specific elimination of LH action does not hamper this process. The backup system, to compensate for eventually disrupted LH action, is provided in the mouse by a complex network of various paracrine activities, as has been demonstrated in other studies (El-Gehani et al. 1998a,b,c, 2000).

It is interesting to compare the completely masculinized phenotype of the neonatal LuRKO mice with phenotype of the humans with completely inactivating LHβ (Weiss et al. 1992) and LHR mutations (Themmen and Huhtaniemi 2000). The one male described with inactivating mutation in the LHβ subunit was normally masculinized at birth but totally lacked the postnatal phase of masculinization. In contrast, males with completely inactivating mutations of the LHR gene have phenotypes with total lack of fetal and postnatal masculinization, i.e. pseudo-hermaphroditism. The explanation for the two different phenotypes is that in the absence of pituitary LH, placental hCG is able to stimulate steroidogenesis of the human fetal Leydig cells (Huhtaniemi 1994), whereas if the LHR is inactivated, neither LH nor hCG are able to stimulate Leydig cell steroidogenesis. It is intriguing that the backup systems for defective gonadotropin production in utero (hCG or paracrine effects) in man and rodent are so different for such a universal developmental event as masculine differentiation.

When the LuRKO and WT male mice were compared in adult age, the total lack of postnatal growth of male genital structures was apparent in the former group. Although all male genital organs had apparently differentiated normally in utero, their growth was totally blocked postnatally (Fig. 1). Testicular descent was also absent, and upon histological examination, the LuRKO testes displayed underdeveloped seminiferous tubules, with sporadic round spermatids being the most advanced form of spermatogenesis. Small and poorly differentiated Leydig cells were present in the interstitium. Because the *hpg* mice are totally devoid of both LH and FSH action, their spermatogenesis stops before meiosis at the pachytene spermatocyte stage. Hence, the progression through meiosis (from pachytene spermatocytes to round spermatids) is apparently stimulated by FSH in the LuRKO testes, which are exposed to normal or even elevated action of this gonadotropin. The fact that full spermatogenesis was not found is either due to the cryptorchid position

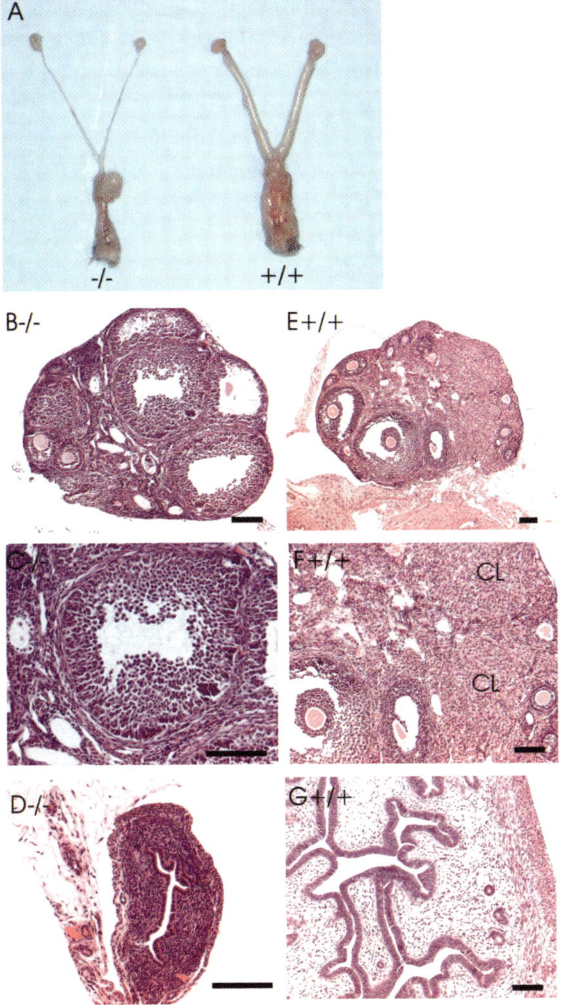

Fig. 2A–G. Morphology and histology of ovaries and genital organs of control WT and homozygous LuRKO female mice. **A** Ovaries, uteri and vagina of a KO and a WT littermate. **B, E** Ovarian histology of a 7-week-old KO and WT mouse. **C, F** As in **B** and **E**, at higher magnification. **D, G** Uterine histology and a KO and WT mouse. *CL*, corpus luteum. *Bar* in panels **B–G**, 100 μm

of the KO testes, insufficient intratesticular testosterone concentration, or both. Androgen replacement therapy of the KO male mice will demonstrate to what extent testicular descent and spermatogenesis can be recovered.

In female (-/-) mice, the age of vaginal opening was delayed by 3–5 days, and the ovaries were about 50% reduced in size and the uteri were significantly thinner (Fig. 2). Ovarian histology showed, conspicuously, relatively normal theca cell layer around the developing follicles (Fig. 2). However, follicular development appeared to stop at the early antral stage, and there were no signs of ovulation or follicular luteinization (Fig. 2). The ovaries of *hpg* and common α-subunit KO mice had follicles up to the preantral stage, which indicated that FSH has an effect on the progression of preantral follicles to early antral stage. The female phenotype of the LuRKO mice is even closer to that of the inactivating human LHR mutations (Themmen and Huhtaniemi 2000). Affected women have normal primary and secondary sex characteristics, increased gonodotropins, and low estrogen and progesterone production. Likewise, suppressed but not absent estrogen production of the LuRKO mice is reflected by presence of granulosa cells in their ovaries, delayed vaginal opening, and hypoplastic uteri. Ovarian histology demonstrates follicles at early stages of development, but no preovulatory follicles or corpora lutea, in agreement with findings on women with inactivating LHR mutations. It was intriguing to note that the progression in follicular development from the early antral to antral and preovulatory stages, in addition to ovulation and luteinization, are LH dependent phenomena, since they also were missing in the KO mice.

No extragonadal phenotypes were found in the LuRKO mice, which speaks against a major role of the recently found ubiquitous LHR expression in nongonadal tissues.

7.5 Conclusions

Our knowledge of the structure and function of LH and LHR has expanded during past years, largely due to the development of molecular biology techniques as well as to the discovery of activating and inactivating mutations of LH and LHR genes in humans. The consequences of human mutations in the LH and its receptor genes strengthened earlier concepts of the main physiological and pathophysiological actions of LH in the ovary and testis. In addition, they have provided more detailed information about numerous less well-known aspects of LH function. These findings have been corroborated by a number of TG and KO mouse models. They allow us to identify directly the specific LH-dependent steps of male and female sexual differentiation and their role in adult gonadal functions. The KO mouse models are very close phenocopies of inactivating mutations of the human LH and LHR genes, and they provide a valuable tool for experimental studies of pathogenesis of this condition.

Acknowledgements. The original studies reviewed in this paper were supported by grants from the Academy of Finland, The Sigrid Jusélius Foundation and The Finnish Cancer Foundation.

References

Cattanach BM, IC, Charlton HM, Chiappa SA, Fink G (1977) Gonadotrophin-releasing hormone deficiency in a mutant mouse with hypogonadism. Nature 269:338–340

Charlton HM (1984) Mouse mutants as models in endocrine research. Q J Exp Physiol 69:655–676

Desjardins C (1981) Endocrine signaling and male reproduction. Biol Reprod 24:1–21

Dierich A, Sairam MR, Monaco L, Fimia GM, Gansmuller A, LeMeur M, Sassone-Corsi P (1998) Impairing follicle-stimulating hormone (FSH) signaling in vivo: targeted disruption of the FSH receptor leads to aberrant gametogenesis and hormonal imbalance. Proc Natl Acad Sci U S A 95:13612–13617

El-Gehani F, Tena-Sempere M, Huhtaniemi I (1998a) Vasoactive intestinal peptide is an important endocrine regulatory factor of fetal rat testicular steroidogenesis. Endocrinology 139:1474–1480

El-Gehani F, Tena-Sempere M, Huhtaniemi I (1998b) Vasoactive intestinal peptide stimulates testosterone production by cultured fetal rat testicular cells. Mol Cell Endocrinol 140:175–178

El-Gehani F, Tena-Sempere M, Huhtaniemi I (2000) Evidence that pituitary adenylate cyclase-activating polypeptide is a potent regulator of fetal rat testicular steroidogenesis. Biol Reprod 63:1482–1489

El-Gehani F, Zhang FP, Pakarinen P, Rannikko A, Huhtaniemi I (1998c) Gonadotropin-independent regulation of steroidogenesis in the fetal rat testis. Biol Reprod 58:116–123

Gharib SD, Wierman ME, Shupnik MA, Chin WW (1990) Molecular biology of the pituitary gonadotropins. Endocr Rev 11:177–199

Huhtaniemi I (1994) Fetal testis–a very special endocrine organ. Eur J Endocrinol 130:25–31

Huhtaniemi IT, Korenbrot CC, Jaffe RB (1977) hCG binding and stimulation of testosterone biosynthesis in the human fetal testis. J Clin Endocrinol Metab 44:963–967

Kendall SK, Samuelson LC, Saunders TL, Wood RI, Camper SA (1995) Targeted disruption of the pituitary glycoprotein hormone alpha-subunit produces hypogonadal and hypothyroid mice. Genes Dev 9:2007–2019

Kremer H, Kraaij R, Toledo SP, Post M, Fridman JB, Hayashida CY, van Reen M, Milgrom E, Ropers HH, Mariman E, et al (1995) Male pseudohermaphroditism due to a homozygous missense mutation of the luteinizing hormone receptor gene. Nat Genet 9:160–164

Kumar TR, Wang Y, Lu N, Matzuk MM (1997) Follicle stimulating hormone is required for ovarian follicle maturation but not male fertility. Nat Genet 15:201–204

Lei ZM, Mishra S, Zou W, Xu B, Foltz M, Li X, Rao CV (2001) Targeted disruption of luteinizing hormone/human chorionic gonadotropin receptor gene. Mol Endocrinol 15:184–200

Mason AJ, Hayflick JS, Zoeller RT, Young WS, 3rd, Phillips HS, Nikolics K, Seeburg PH (1986) A deletion truncating the gonadotropin-releasing hormone gene is responsible for hypogonadism in the hpg mouse. Science 234: 1366–1371

Mason AJ, Pitts SL, Nikolics K, Szonyi E, Wilcox JN, Seeburg PH, Stewart TA (1986) The hypogonadal mouse: reproductive functions restored by gene therapy. Science 234:1372–1378

O'Shaughnessy PJ, Baker P, Sohnius U, Haavisto AM, Charlton HM, Huhtaniemi I (1998) Fetal development of Leydig cell activity in the mouse is independent of pituitary gonadotroph function. Endocrinology 139: 1141–1146

Richards JS (1994) Hormonal control of gene expression in the ovary. Endocr Rev 15:725–751

Richards JS (2001) Perspective: the ovarian follicle – a perspective in 2001. Endocrinology 142:2184–2193

Richards JS, Fitzpatrick SL, Clemens JW, Morris JK, Alliston T, Sirois J (1995) Ovarian cell differentiation: a cascade of multiple hormones, cellular signals, and regulated genes. Recent Prog Horm Res 50:223–254

Saez JM (1994) Leydig cells: endocrine, paracrine, and autocrine regulation. Endocr Rev 15:574–626

Segaloff DL, Ascoli M (1993) The lutropin/choriogonadotropin receptor ... 4 years later. Endocr Rev 14:324–347

Tena-Sempere M, Huhtaniemi IT (1999) Gonadotropin receptors. In: Molecular Biology in Reproductive Medicine. Eds Frauser BCMJ, Rutherford AJ, Strauss JF, III, Van Steirteghem A. New York, Parthenon Publishing, pp 165–200

Themmen APN, Huhtaniemi IT (2000) Mutations of gonadotropins and gonadotropin receptors: elucidating the physiology and pathophysiology of pituitary-gonadal function. Endocr Rev 21:551–583

Weiss J, Axelrod L, Whitcomb RW, Harris PE, Crowley WF, Jameson JL (1992) Hypogonadism caused by a single amino acid substitution in the beta subunit of luteinizing hormone. N Engl J Med 326:179–183

Zhang FP, Poutanen M, Wilbertz J, Huhtaniemi I (2001) Normal prenatal but arrested postnatal sexual development of luteinizing hormone receptor knockout (LuRKO) mice. Mol Endocrinol 15:172–183

Zhang, FP, Rannikko AS, Manna PR, Fraser HM, Huhtaniemi IT (1997) Cloning and functional expression of the luteinizing hormone receptor complementary deoxyribonucleic acid from the marmoset monkey testis: absence of sequences encoding exon 10 in other species. Endocrinology 138:2481–2490.

8 Analysing Differential Gene Expression in the Testis

R. Ivell, A.-N. Spiess

8.1 Introduction

The testis in mammals has to perform three principal functions. Firstly, it is the place where the male gametes are generated from undifferentiated stem cells (spermatogonia), through regulated processes of proliferation and reduction division. There is a continuous production of haploid nuclei enclosed within highly specialized transport systems (spermatozoa) capable of conveying the haploid nucleus through a relatively inimical environment (the female tract) to undergo specific nuclear fusion with the female gamete. Secondly, the testis is the organ producing the male sex steroid hormone, testosterone (and other hormones) in a regulated fashion (e.g. negative feedback through the pituitary-gonadal axis) to provide an appropriate gender-specific environment for the correct development and management of other organ systems. Thirdly, the testis is the principal organ of evolution, where small changes in the inherited genome are tolerated (encouraged) during spermatogenesis in order to provide individual variation and hence potential species adaptation. This function requires an organ-specific regulation of DNA replication, recombination and repair.

The attainment of these three functions is a resultant of profound and continuing differentiation processes, not only through embryonic development and puberty, but ongoing throughout life with the persistent generation of (in humans) ca. 100 million spermatozoa per day up to old age. While in spermatozoa we have an example of a cell type with high cell turnover, the testis is host to other cells (e.g. Leydig cells) which, after puberty, are calculated to maintain their function and individual existence almost for the lifetime of the organism.

Given this complexity and variety in functional expression, it is not surprising that this is reflected by high complexity also at the genotypic level. As far as we can judge from the still limited information from the various genome projects, the testis is an organ with a high degree of organ- and cell-type specific gene expression, both in terms of individual genes as well as in terms of transcript variants (alternative splicing).

8.2 Holistic Assessment of Testis Gene Expression

For a variety of reasons, scientific, philosophical and aesthetic, the testis has been a subject of visual analysis for many decades. Implicit in these anatomical studies is the need to have a method of assessment of testicular function which is at once both analytical and holistic. Still today, most of what we know about the testis derives from morphological analysis of individual cell components. The problem is that apart from a few molecules, acting as surrogates for cell function, we have very little knowledge of the molecular basis for what we see under the microscope. For the plethora of strange and wonderful structures and organelles imaged from the healthy or from the diseased organ, possibly only a few percent can be associated with a specific biochemistry of component molecules. What has long been required for andrology is a method that allows a holistic appraisal of testicular function at the molecular level.

Before going into detail on the various molecular approaches that have been tried, we need first to appreciate the variable cellularity of the

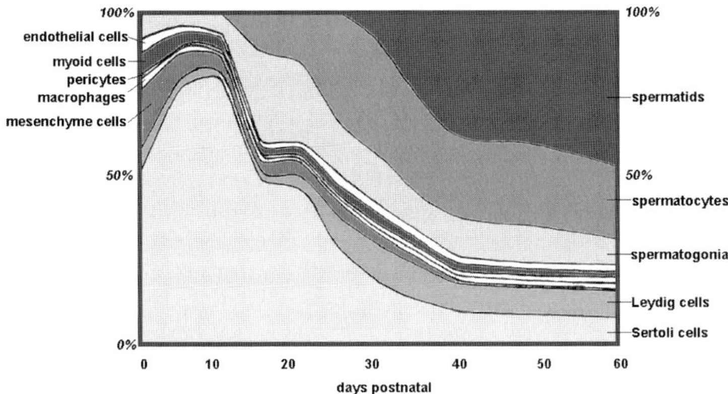

Fig. 1. Estimated proportions of different cell types (percent of all cell nuclei) at different postnatal times during the development of the rat testis. Data were extrapolated from results presented in Hardy et al. (1989), Yang et al. (1990) and Gondos and Berndtson (1993)

testis, which will be represented in any gene expression profile. In the interstitial space, there are Leydig cells, precursor mesenchyme cells, macrophages, other lymphoid cells, vascular endothelial cells, vascular smooth muscle cells, and the so-called co-cells or pericytes. The seminiferous tubules comprise all pre- and post-meiotic germ cells, Sertoli cells, peritubular myoid cells, as well as a similar complement of vascular and connective tissue cells to the interstitium. Finally, there are the cells of the specialized regions, such as the rete testis or the tunica albuginea. Then one has to consider that most of these cell types will exist in several different states of differentiation. Thus each individual cell type will contribute to the holistic pattern of testis gene expression corresponding to its individual functional/phenotypic status at any one time.

Equally important, however, is the fact that the proportional contribution made by any one cell type will change depending upon the developmental or disease status of the testis. Figure 1 represents a collation of morphometric results documenting the number of cell nuclei (as units of gene expression) for different cell types through postnatal development of the rat testis. Thus, a Sertoli cell-specific mRNA may appear to be more highly expressed in the prepubertal rat testis, compared to the adult testis, not because it is indeed upregulated in individual Sertoli cells, but simply because these make up a much greater proportion of total testicular volume before spermatogenesis has begun. Similarly, while in tubules from a day 20 rat testis spermatogonia comprise approximately 65% of all germ cells, the remainder being developing spermatocytes, on day 40, spermatogonia comprise only about 16%, spermatocytes 33%, and now spermatids make up half the germ cell complement (Yang et al. 1990). Correspondingly, any post-meiotically expressed gene will appear to be massively up-regulated in day 40–60 testis samples compared to earlier times.

The Human Genome Project currently predicts a total number of genes in the human genome of about 35,000, though the figure may become higher because of the ineffectiveness of current bioinformatic algorithms to identify all expressed genes in the genome. It is estimated that of these, some 5,000–10,000 will be expressed in a specific cell-type, and possibly 20,000–25,000 will be expressed in any one tissue. Based on current EST (expressed sequence tag) information, there appears to be an average of 7 different gene transcripts for any single gene. These alternative transcripts may have different 5′ untranslated regions (UTR), which do not influence the open reading frame (ORF) and hence the encoded protein, but do belie a probably different transcription start-site, and hence regulatory region (promoter) for the gene in question. Alternatively, there may be transcripts with different 3′ UTRs due to alternative polyadenylation, which again do not affect the encoded protein, but may influence the rate of degradation and hence turnover of the specific mRNA. Finally, alternative transcripts may be the result of alternative exon splicing, particularly within the ORF, such that different protein products may result. One gene, for example that for C/EBPß, can give rise to either stimulatory (LAP) or inhibitory (LIP) transcription factors, depending upon which start methionine is used for translation (Descombes and Schibler 1991).

At the protein level, variability is much greater. Not only can alternative transcripts give rise to different ORFs, but a single ORF can vary in its expressed phenotype, depending upon the use of the translational start methionine, or whether the protein is post-translationally modified by proteolysis, esterification, glycosylation, phosphorylation, sulfatation, isoprenylation, palmitoylation, etc. Each of these modifications can be cell-type specific and very variable. So, for example, for the epididymis-specific form of the sperm surface antigen CD52 at least 51 different glycosylaton variants have been characterized (Schröter et al. 2000). Also, while often true, it is definitely not consistent that mRNAs and their encoded proteins are regulated in parallel. A common mRNA may be translated very poorly, whereas a rare mRNA could be translated with high efficiency.

This knowledge needs to be considered in choosing an approach for a holistic appraisal of testis molecular biology. For a modern gene chip (DNA microarray) with target cDNA (e.g. EST) sequences recognizing most alternative transcript variants of any one gene, then 20,000 different gene targets could reflect most of the genes expressed in the testis. This is pragmatically manageable, but would provide no information on alternative transcript usage, nor on their protein products. The use of oligonucleotide arrays is an improvement both technically (see later) and because these can be designed to distinguish between different alternative transcripts from the same gene. To cover all possible transcripts in the testis, however, would necessitate 7×20,000=140,000 different target molecules on the chip, and this would still not say anything about the proteins expressed. The current alternative to this kind of transcriptome analysis is proteome analysis. But when one considers that the proteome of a single cell probably encompasses more than 100,000 different protein variants, then even the most sophisticated 2-dimensional electrophoresis or LC-LC separation system will need to be restricted to specific subsets of proteins, especially where an organ is to be investigated such as the testis. Successful examples of proteome application for the testis have been provided by the laboratories of John Herr and Charles Pineau, where either cell types (e.g. ejaculated spermatozoa or spermatogonia) have been focussed upon, or their subcellular components (e.g. vectorially labelled surface antigens) (Naaby-Hansen et al. 1997; Guillaume et al. 2001). Possibly one of the best (and oldest) examples of successful proteome application was the discovery by Douglas Stocco of the StAR (steroidogenic acute regulatory) protein in the mitochondria of Leydig cells (Clark et al. 1994).

8.3 Analysis of Differential Gene Expression in the Testis

When we consider what would be the ideal holistic approach to assessing gene expression in a tissue like the testis, then one possibility would be a DNA chip whereon all genes known to be expressed in the testis are represented, and then making use of oligonucleotide probes so that also different transcript variants can be assessed. As mentioned before, such a chip would be very large (ca. 140,000 targets), and prohibitively expensive to produce for such a limited market as the testis. Also, most of the bioinformatic data required are still not available for the design of appropriate oligonucleotides. But even if such a chip were feasible, then it is evident to most scientists that the informational content of the chip would be a lot less than its potential capacity. The reason for this is that just because a gene is expressed does not mean that it is physiologically relevant in the context in which the DNA chip is to be used. Probably more than half the genes will represent housekeeping functions which are neither cell-type specific nor physiologically relevant in the context of the scientific questions being asked. A further substantial proportion of the transcripts will be below the level of practical detection (see later). Thus, the DNA chip could be reduced substantially in dimensions, if it were possible to have only transcripts represented, which were informationally relevant in a physiological sense, and which could be physically detected.

Our Hamburg research group, like many others, has pursued a variety of approaches to optimize both these aspects of specific testicular gene expression. In the present review we shall look firstly at the approaches possible with which to define physiologically relevant genes. Then we shall look at aspects of hybridization theory in order to determine the physical and informational cutoff for such a holistic approach.

8.4 Bioinformatics and Datamining

A consequence of the Human Genome Project is the creation of a variety of excellent genome and transcriptome databases. Whilst the genome databases are valuable for checking and completion of sequences, and for determination of genomic parameters, the transcriptome databases are invaluable sources of information on tissue-specific gene expression.

These databases comprise two sorts of sequence, the EST (expressed sequence tag) representing a partial sequence (usually 3′ end) of cDNA clones selected randomly from a particular cDNA library, and more recently the full-length mRNA sequences, compiled from different ESTs and other information. There are several excellent resources available, which can be very helpful for checking the structure (splice form) and sequence of a transcript, and its identity, where known. Less helpful are the annotations for the sequences, where these are based not on detailed expression data in the form of organ-specific publications, but solely on the source of the cDNA library from which the sequences were derived. One of the earliest of these was the Soares human testis library, based on a commercial bacteriophage library. Whilst neither subtracted nor normalized, this library had been amplified so that shorter cDNAs were probably over-represented and, as in all such early cDNA libraries, longer transcripts are under-represented. Being a conventional library, EST sequences should theoretically occur in the database at a frequency more or less corresponding to their expression level in the tissue concerned. This is the basis for the in silico northerns that can be performed just using the information in the databases. However, just because an EST sequence is derived from a testis cDNA library does not imply testis expression in a physiological sense. The testis comprises many cell types, and on a statistical basis, virtually any gene could be expressed somewhere at a very low level, without this meaning anything physiologically for the cell. Similarly, the same gene might be expressed at a much higher level in another tissue, but this information is not included in the database. Thus the notation 'testis' attached to such an EST clone can be very misleading. The RIKEN mouse testis library is in this context more useful since it is large and is being compiled into full-length transcripts where sufficient independent clones are available to make this possible. Thus, in theory such transcript information can be collated into a list of testis-expressed transcripts, with information on relative frequency and structure. Such a list, however, still does not tell us much about the physiological relevance of the transcripts, or whether they should be included on our idealized DNA chip.

An alternative approach has been to datamine both gene and literature databases, thus selecting genes for which there is validated physiological (expression) information. This is the basis for the TestisBank of the University of Münster research group in Germany (http://medweb.uni-muenster.de/TestisBank/) and for the MRG database from the USA (http://mouse.genetics.washington.edu/; Braun and Cassen 2001). These are of necessity still very small. Thus at present, it would appear that a datamining approach to select transcripts appropriate for a testis-specific DNA chip is still some way off.

8.5 Differential cDNA Cloning

There are a number of testis transcript sequences in the databases which have not come from large-scale EST projects, but from individual differential cloning projects. These are sporadic sequences, where usually only a few differentially expressed genes have been detected in any one project, indicating that the methods applied are far from exhaustive. This is true for almost all differential cloning techniques being used, where it is evident that the authors are generally grateful to publish results on a few cDNA clones which are novel and fulfil the requirements for differential expression. It is important to understand the limitations of these techniques in order to evaluate the usefulness of the results.

8.5.1 Differential (Plus/Minus) Screening of cDNA Libraries

Screening by plaque hybridization of non-confluent cDNA libraries in bacteriophage using complex cDNA probes comprising all transcripts in their natural proportions from one tissue compared with a similar complex probe from another tissue, or another developmental state, has proved very successful for identifying commonly expressed genes (Fig. 2). In earlier studies comparing testis with a pool of other tissues, a handful of genes such as the protamines, LDH-C or TCP-1 were discovered (e.g. Kleene et al. 1983; Willison et al. 1986; Thomas et al. 1989; Höög 1991). These are very frequently expressed genes found predominantly in spermatids, which are not only the most frequent cell type in the mature testis, but are also biosynthetically very active. Similar studies were carried out for the epididymis, where again this approach allowed the discovery of several new genes, the majority of which proved to encode major secretory products of the epididymal epithelium (Kirchhoff et al. 1990; Ivell et al. 1998).

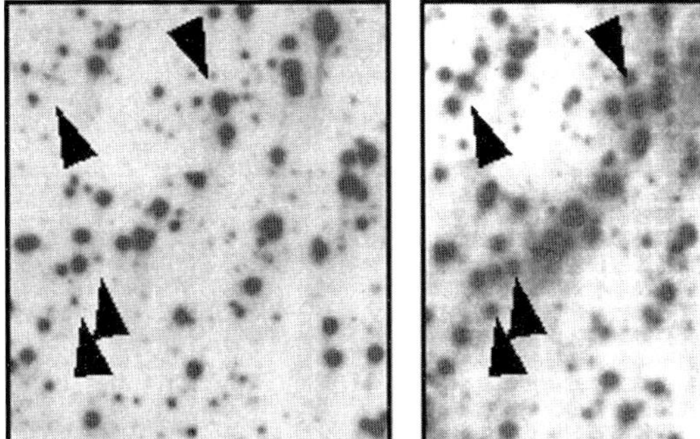

Fig. 2. Differential (plus/minus) screening of a human epididymal cDNA library in bacteriophage lambda (Kirchhoff et al. 1990). Duplicate plaque lifts were hybridized to radiolabelled complex cDNA probes derived from HeLa cells (*left panel*) or human epididymis (*right panel*). Clones differentially expressed in the epididymis are indicated by *arrowheads*. (Courtesy of Dr. C. Kirchhoff)

The limitations of this approach are firstly, that clones to be screened must be non-confluent. In practical terms, given limited amounts of probe, time and handling capacity, not more than about 100,000 independent cDNA clones can be screened successfully. There is a formula (Eq. 1) which defines the number of clones in a conventional (non-normalized, non-subtracted) library which need to be screened in order statistically to obtain a 99% probability of finding a particular gene clone. According to this formula screening of 100,000 clones would limit the statistical detection limit of the system to transcripts with a frequency greater than 0.005%.

$$N = \frac{I_n\,(1\text{-}P)}{I_n\,(1\text{-}n)}$$

where
- N=number of cDNA clones screened
- P=the desired probability (e.g. 0.99)
- n=fractional proportion of the total mRNA population that a single mRNA represents
- and l_n=natural logarithm

Table 1. Distribution of gene transcripts in a tissue

Tissue	Number of different mRNAs	Abundance (molecules/cell)	Average mRNA prevalence (%of total mRNA)	Category
Mouse liver	9	12,000	2.5%	Abundant
	700	300	0.06%	Moderate
	11,500	15	0.003%	Rare
Chick oviduct	1	100,000	52.5%	
	7	4,000	2.1%	
	12,500	5	0.002%	

In Table 1 are listed figures for the relative frequency of different transcripts in two well characterized tissues, the mouse liver and the chicken oviduct. The testis is probably more complex than either of these (i.e. closer to 20,000 total genes expressed) and in the distribution of abundance categories intermediate between the two. Accordingly, transcripts with an individual frequency below 0.005% should comprise approximately 97% of all genes expressed. Statistically, therefore, these transcripts are unlikely to be detected in a differential screening approach.

There is another limitation, however, in the screening of cDNA clones using complex probes, which is also valid for the interrogation of DNA chips and other DNA-arrays. This is a function of the kinetic parameters of nucleic acid hybridization (Maniatis et al. 1982; Hames and Higgins 1985). Firstly, we need to consider temperature. The melting temperature (T_m) of a DNA hybrid is the temperature at which complementary strands are 50% hybridized, and depends on the nucleotide composition of the DNA. For long fragments (>100 bp):

$$(DNA > 100\ bp)$$
$$T_m = 81.5°C - 16.6(\log_{10}[Na^+]) + 0.41\ (\%G+C) - 0.63\ (\%formamide) - (600/N) \tag{2}$$

where N is the length of the DNA in base pairs.

For oligonucleotides (DNA <100 bp) the T_m can be approximated as follows:

(DNA <100 bp)

$$T_m=(\Sigma G+C\times4°C)+(\Sigma A+T\times2°C) \tag{3}$$

In general, hybridization temperatures are chosen to be a few degrees ($<20°C$) below the T_m to encourage more rapid hybridization, but too low a temperature increases mismatching and hence false-positive hybridization. DNA-DNA hybridization in the context of bacteriophage plaque screening or screening of DNA chips and miniarrays follows pseudo first-order kinetics, since the target DNA in the solid phase is generally in a large excess over that in the liquid phase (probe). Under these conditions, then the proportion of hybrid formed is an exponential function of time:

$$[hybrid]=[probe](1-e^{-k[target]t}) \tag{4}$$

Under typical hybridization conditions, the time (t) to reach $C_0t_{1/2}$ (i.e. when half the probe is in the form of a hybrid with its target DNA) is given by:

$$t\ (hours)=1/(\mu g\ probe)\times(complexity\ in\ kb)/5\times(volume\ in\ ml)/5 \tag{5}$$

If we take 3 days (72 h) as the maximum practicable hybridization time, a hybridization volume of 10 ml and a probe complexity (length) of 500 bp, then the minimum probe amount required to reach $C_0t_{1/2}$ is 3 ng. This is for a simple single-stranded cDNA probe. For a complex probe made by reverse transcription of a pool of poly(A)-enriched RNA, where, for example, a total of 1 µg of labelled cDNA can be made and used in a hybridization, this means that only mRNAs can be detected (50% hybridization) which occur at a transcript frequency of greater than 0.3%. In practise, we try to improve on these figures by using smaller effective hybridization volumes through the application of volume-reducing agents such as dextrin, and by accepting hybridization proportions much less than 50%. Even so, we and others have shown in practise that cDNA clones cannot be detected using complex cDNA probes for transcripts which have expression frequencies below 0.01–0.005% (Ivell et al. 1998). Referring again to Table 1, shows that this second limitation also restricts gene detection to those transcripts in the moderate – abundant classes, which include, besides a few tissue-specific secretory products or structural proteins, mostly housekeeping molecules found in all cells, and therefore not of informational relevance in the context of testis science.

8.5.2 Subtractive (Differential) cDNA Cloning

One approach that has been developed to overcome this problem of sensitivity has been to subtract the complex mRNA pools of the plus or minus tissues prior to hybridization, and then to amplify the resulting subtracted probe by PCR to attain a high concentration for hybridization. A variant of this (subtractive cloning) uses the resultant subtractive probe not for hybridization, but to construct a subtracted cDNA library. The subtraction procedure comprises essentially three steps. Firstly, one of the pools of mRNA is converted to the complementary (antisense) single-strand cDNA, followed by elimination of the mRNA from which it was programmed. In the second step this antisense cDNA is hybridized with the mRNA (sense) from the second tissue. This is a liquid phase hybridization and hence follows second-order kinetics. In the third step, the double-stranded RNA-DNA hybrids are separated from the single stranded mRNA and cDNA molecules. After removal of mRNA the remaining single-stranded cDNA molecules are available for PCR amplification to make either probes or libraries. Because of the second-order kinetics, this resulting cDNA pool will not only contain differentially expressed transcripts, but also transcripts whose original frequency was below the concentration for effective hybridization. Thus, although this method allows the advantage of probe amplification or making a preselected differential cDNA library, it will still include a lot of transcripts which are not differentially expressed, but simply of low frequency. The truly differentially expressed genes will be limited to those of a relatively high frequency, which is high enough above the non-specific background to be readily detected. In practise, this method offers approximately an order of magnitude more sensitivity compared to the older differential screening approach, but not more. We have successfully used this method to identify several novel and important testis-specific genes (Pusch et al. 1996a, 1996b).

8.5.3 Differential Display RT-PCR and Related Techniques

Differential display (DD)RT-PCR potentially is a wonderful method for the holistic expression of all transcripts expressed in a cell or tissue type (Liang and Pardee 1992; Ozaki et al. 1996; Catalano et al. 1997; Hansis et al. 1998). By directly comparing the patterns obtained from two discrete tissues, differences in individual gene expression can be easily detected, and the gene products cloned and identified. The great advantage of this method compared to the previous ones is that it is independent of the original concentration of transcripts, and hence even rare transcripts can potentially be detected (>0.0002%; Ozaki et al. 1996). Nevertheless, there are significant limitations. Firstly, to be comprehensive (i.e. fulfil our demands for a holistic method) it requires at least 324 independent PCR reactions for each sample, employing all the combinations of PCR primers recommended in the diverse publications on the method. Even then, these primers do not represent all possible transcript sequences, but rely on a significant degree of mismatch occurring at the selected primer hybridization temperature which is as a rule considerably below the T_m for the different oligonucleotides. Secondly, the final products are 'displayed' on large sequencing gels, selecting the PCR products which fall within the range 100–500 bp. Randomly, with the chosen primers and assuming temperature-dependent mismatching, such fragments should occur for the majority of long transcripts. However, shorter transcripts are decidedly selected against. So, for example, in an exercise to apply DDRT-PCR to clone novel epididymis-specific gene transcripts, we found that over half of the already known and specifically expressed transcripts for small secretory proteins a priori would not be detected by this method (K. Ellerbrock and R. Ivell, unpublished), which is clearly prejudiced towards long transcripts.

There is an inevitable compromise in this method between hybridization specificity and mismatching (comprehensiveness), controlled by the choice of primer hybridization temperature. In an extensive series of control experiments (Hansis et al. 1998) we found that a reasonable balance could be obtained, at the cost, however, of differentially expressed bands on the resulting gels containing the products of more than one gene transcript. As a rule we found that each band contained up to 5 different products, the majority of which would not be differentially expressed and hence created an inevitable false-positive background band intensity. Thus, differentially expressed products were obtained only where the differential transcript was expressed at a high level, or where, by chance, the DDRT-PCR product was not smothered by other comigrating products.

Finally, there is an inevitable degree of experimental variability, such that it is to be recommended that all experiments are repeated several times, and only where a band repeatedly appears to be differentially expressed, is it worth pursuing this product. Altogether, this method has the potential to offer a comprehensive (holistic) picture of differential gene expression in a given tissue. However, considerable practical difficulties appear to limit its usefulness, and the majority of successful publications using this method report on only isolated gene products or groups of gene products.

Recently, as a response to the technical difficulties of conventional DDRT-PCR, several more simple alternatives have appeared on the market. These make use either of a restricted selection of primers, often combining the reverse transcription primer with the amplification primer (e.g. RAP-PCR; Stratagene, La Jolla, CA), and offer at best a transcript 'fingerprint' of a tissue. There is no claim to comprehensiveness. An interesting alternative, is the application of a Taq1 cleavage step, following cDNA synthesis (e.g. RFDD-PCR; Display Systems, Copenhagen). This restriction enzyme cuts the genome randomly every 400–500 bases at the sequence TCGA, and hence theoretically should cleave all cDNAs into a transcript-specific, but diverse selection of fragments of appropriate size for display on a sequencing gel. Unfortunately, being a statistical method, there are approximately 10% of all cDNAs in the international database which do not possess a Taq1 cleavage site; this proportion is increased for short gene transcripts (<1 kb), which as in conventional DDRT-PCR are thus heavily weighted against.

8.5.4 Subtractive Suppression RT-PCR

The aim of all of these procedures is to identify genes which are informationally relevant for testis physiology. Informational relevance has been defined as tissue (testis)-specific expression, though equally one could use a hormonally stimulated (normal adult) versus an unstimulated (immature, antiandrogen- or GnRH agonist/antagonist-treated) organ, or testes from wild type vs mutant animals (e.g. w/w^v azoospermic mice). Genes which are differentially expressed between the two tissues are unlikely to include informationally redundant genes, such as those encoding housekeeping enzymes or structural proteins. Of the 20,000 genes which are probably expressed in the testis, only about 25%, or 5,000, are likely to be informationally important in the context of specific testis function. This is still a much larger number than those which have altogether been identified by the various cloning strategies described so far.

A new technique promises to be much more effective in identifying all the informationally relevant genes. Subtractive suppression (SS)RT-PCR (Diatchenko et al. 1996) is a PCR-based technique, which has several added advantages over the previous techniques. Firstly, the mutual hybridization step to distinguish similarity from difference by separation of single- from double-stranded nucleic acids, occurs following digestion with the restriction enzyme RsaI allowing more rapid and homogeneous kinetics with most fragments being about 500 bp long. Secondly, there are several 'PCR-tricks' employed which not only encourage amplification of the differentially expressed transcript copies, but deliberately suppress (hence the name) transcripts shared in common between the two transcript pools. The result is a pool of transcript copies which are both differentially expressed and at the same time normalized, i.e. not present at concentrations corresponding to the original expression frequency in the tissue. The resulting pool of transcript cDNA copies has therefore very low redundancy (and thus high information content) and can be amplified further by PCR, and cloned into an appropriate vector to make a very useful and specific cDNA library.

In the original publications, testis RNA was compared with a pool of RNA from a variety of non-testis tissues (Diatchenko et al. 1996; Jin et al. 1997). In these and most subsequent publications using this technique, several hundred different and specific cDNA clones were generated, representing a major increase over earlier methods. However, this is still a long way short of the 5,000 independent clones which would allow a comprehensive overview of testis physiology.

We have recently begun systematically to optimize the different steps involved in this procedure. Firstly, we have improved the first-strand cDNA synthesis by including various co-solutes, and have thereby in-

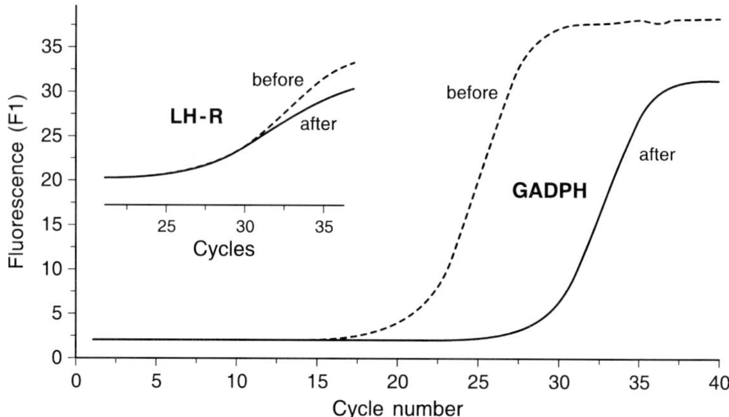

Fig. 3. Quantitative real-time (LightCycler) PCR analysis for a rare (LH-receptor) and a common transcript (GAPDH) before and after the common subtraction/normalization process employed in SSRT-PCR. Whereas for the rare transcript there is no effective change in the 'crossing-point', for the common transcript, the 'crossing-point' has been shifted to the right by about 9 cycles, equivalent to a 2^9-(=512-)fold reduction in relative amount

creased both yield, and especially length of resulting cDNA clones (Spiess and Ivell 2002). Now, even very long transcripts (e.g. clathrin, 14.4 kb) are efficiently represented in the starting cDNA pools. Secondly, for effective hybridization of differentially expressed transcripts, it is important that the products of the first PCR amplification still retain all transcripts in the same proportion to one another as in the original hybridized mixture. To optimize these conditions, we monitored the linear amplification phase of a common testis transcript (that for RLF/INSL3) using real-time PCR (LightCycler; Roche, Mannheim, Germany) and stopped the PCR reaction just before this became non-linear. We can safely assume, therefore, that this and all less frequent transcripts are still in the linear phase of amplification, and hence have retained their subtracted relative frequency after this PCR step. Finally, we have monitored and optimized the subsequent suppression and normalization steps, also using real-time PCR, for a typical common transcript (for GAPDH) and a rare transcript (for the LH receptor). Comparing the amounts of the two transcripts before and after the normalization/suppression step shows a large difference in concentration for the GAPDH, but no difference for the LH receptor transcripts (Fig. 3).

In this example, using rat testis, cloning of the resulting differential cDNA pool has led to a library of approximately 5,000 cDNA clones. Randomly testing these cDNA clones by restriction digestion showed firstly that they were all different, i.e. non-redundant. Sequencing of these clones verified this, and also indicated that whilst some corresponded to known testis-specific genes, the majority were either unannotated or simply not represented in the international databases at all. Thus, this method is not only capable of generating a large number of testis-specific cDNA clones, but it confirms what many of us have suspected, that the testis expresses many genes which are either still not yet characterized, or still completely novel. We are currently arraying all these cDNA clones for further characterization of expression patterns.

8.6 Application of DNA Microarrays (DNA Chips)

The development of DNA microarray (DNA chip) technology in the last few years has been dramatic and many excellent review articles have recently been published, particularly concerning their bioinformatic interpretation (e.g. Hess et al. 2001). Less is discussed concerning the practicabilities of their application. Whereas arrayed cDNA clones on nylon filters suffer the same restrictions in sensitivity as replica filters of bacteriophage clones (see above), the smaller dimensions of DNA chips already imply smaller probe volumes and hence up to 100-fold increased relative probe concentration. This allows us theoretically to detect transcripts present in complex cDNA probes at frequencies of <0.0001%, i.e. in the range of rare transcripts, such as those for many signal transduction molecules and transcription factors.

Such probes nevertheless require as starting material several micrograms of poly(A)-enriched mRNA, which for some cells or tissues (e.g. primary cultures of Sertoli cells or Percoll-enriched germ cells) is a prohibitively high amount. One way out of this problem is to make use of PCR-amplified probes, whereby there is considerable risk that the amplification could give rise to a distortion of the relative transcript frequency within each probe. As explained above for the first PCR step of the SSRT-PCR, provided one can monitor that the PCR reaction remains in the linear amplification phase for a common gene product, then probe amplification can both increase sensitivity of detection and allow much smaller amounts of mRNA to be used. When using amplification protocols it is important to monitor such distortion effects through the use of several different constitutive gene targets which should not vary between different experimental procedures. Experience with the first generation of DNA chips which are commercially available shows that there is still a high signal variability, even between chips using the same source of mRNA as probe. Part of this variation due to hybridization or between-chip fluctuations can be overcome by mixing plus and minus probes derived from different sources and synthesized in the presence of different fluorophores, and using this mixture to hybridize to a single DNA chip. The resulting signals are then analysed for both intensity and emitted wave-length, from which the relative proportions of the individual transcripts in the original mixtures can be calculated. Nevertheless, there is still a need for numerous repetitions of experiments and statistical analyses on individual hybridization spots, before a clear statement about up- or down-regulation of a particular gene can be made.

Whilst these practical issues are mostly soluble through the use of appropriate kits, statistical repetition, and closely monitored controls, two important issues need to be considered. Firstly, current DNA chip technology is very expensive. Individual commercial DNA chips cost between US$ 500 and 5,000 each, and can be sensibly used only once. DNA chip scanners cost between US$ 35,000 and 100,000. Analysis software and bioinformatics support should also be considered. Thus for a validated experiment with sufficient replicates for reliable statistical analysis, this inevitably requires either substantial subsidy through a government or university resource centre or a company, or interaction with a DNA chip provider.

The second very important issue is the relevance of the DNA chips available for the physiological question that is being posed. To date, almost all DNA chips are making use of mined information from the databases, and for commercial reasons are tailored to specific tissues, species or functions (e.g. signal transduction, oncogenes and cancer, rat liver, human prostate, etc). For those of us studying the testis, the use of these DNA chips, whilst helpful, will be a long way from being comprehensive, i.e. fulfilling our goal of a holistic molecular equivalent of the histological section, simply because so many of the genes we would be interested in are either not present or not 'visible' in the databases.

8.6.1 The Hamburg Concept

In Hamburg we are working towards the development of a new generation of DNA chips. By applying the SSRT-PCR technology we are creating small (ca. 5,000 clones) differential cDNA libraries comprising sets of clones of high informational relevance. These are being tailored for specific model systems and physiologies; so, for example, we are making testis-specific libraries for the human, marmoset monkey and rat. From our preliminary studies we can assume that these will include a large number of novel (unannotated) gene transcripts which would not be present on any currently available commercial DNA chip. After preliminary validation, these libraries are being sequenced and arrayed on DNA chips, initially as denatured, double-stranded PCR products. Whilst less sensitive, such double-stranded DNA targets will allow a preliminary characterization of the DNA chips to distinguish cDNA clones which are informationally relevant (e.g. vary through puberty, or under pharmacological or pathological perturbation, or are above detection limits). The preliminary information from such studies will then be used in the production of a follow-up generation of DNA chips. This subsequent generation will make use of such experimental findings together with information from the literature (where available), to create an oligonucleotide chip, where we can take account also of genes which were not present in our libraries, but should have been, and of differential transcripts for the same gene, where this is known. The use of oligonucleotides as targets has several advantages. As 50- or 70-mers, they can be designed to avoid any cross-hybridization between related genes, and yet maintain a constant T_m for equivalent hybridization efficiency. There appears to be a lower background hybridization noise for oligonucleotides, as opposed to PCR products, and hence this allows for increased detection sensitivity of specific hybridization signals. And, as oligonucleotides, they can be designed to be very transcript specific, thus taking account of known transcript variants. Clearly, for an academic institution this is a project of epic proportions. However, because we are starting from a physiological question (tissue-specific gene expression) and already at an early stage are methodologically limiting the genes of interest to those which are highly relevant (ca. 5,000 cDNA clones per tissue), the project remains manageable. Much will depend on collaboration with the research community to help us identify and validate genes of interest, especially for the construction of our second generation of DNA chips.

Acknowledgements. We should especially like to thank the Deutsche Forschungsgemeinschaft for research support for this project (Iv7/4–2 and Iv7/10–1), and the German Federal Ministry of Education and Research (BMBF) for an infrastructure grant. We should also like to acknowledge the many colleagues who have participated over the years in building up our knowledge-base on testis-specific gene expression, and in particular Nadine Müller, Marga Balvers, Wolfgang Pusch, Kerstin Ellerbrock and Christoph Hansis, as well as our partners in the DFG Confocal Research Group on 'The Male Gamete' with the University of Münster.

References

Braun RE and Cassen V (2001) Virtual reproductive genetics: applying functional genomics and bioinformatics to research on male reproduction. Biol Reprod 64 (Suppl.1) 84.

Catalano RD, Vlad M and Kennedy RC (1997) Differential display to identify and isolate novel genes expressed during spermatogenesis. Mol Hum Reprod 3: 215–221.

Clark BJ, Wells J, King SR and Stocco DM (1994) The purification, cloning and expression of a novel luteinizing hormone-induced mitochondrial protein in MA-10 mouse Leydig tumor cells. Characterization of the steroidogenic acute regulatory protein (StAR). J Biol Chem 269: 28314–28322.

Descombes P and Schibler U (1991) A liver-enriched transcriptional activator protein, LAP, and a transcriptional inhibitory protein, LIP, are translated from the same mRNA. Cell 67: 569–579.

Diatchenko L, Lau YC, Campbell AP, Chenchik A, Moqadam F, Huang B, Lukyanov S, Lukyanov K, Gurskaya N, Sverdlov ED and Siebert PD (1996) Suppression subtractive hybridization: a method for generating differentially regulated or tissue-specific cDNA probes and libraries. Proc Natl Acad Sci USA, 93: 6025-6030.

Gondos B and Berndston WE (1993) Postnatal and pubertal development. In: The Sertoli cell (Russell LD and Griswold MD, eds.). Cache River Press, Clearwater, FL.

Guillaume E, Pineau C, Evrard B, Dupaix A, Moertz E, Sanchez JC, Hochstrasser DF and Jegou B. (2001) Cellular distribution of translationally controlled tumor protein in rat and human testes. Proteomics 1: 880–889.

Hames BD and Higgins SJ (eds.) (1985) Nucleic acid hybridization: a practical approach. IRL Press, Oxford.

Hansis C, Jähner D, Spiess AN, Boettcher K and Ivell R (1998) The gene for the Alzheimer-associated ß-amyloid-binding protein (ERAB) is differentially expressed in the testicular Leydig cells of the azoospermic w/w^v mouse. Eur J Biochem 258: 53–60.

Hardy MP, Zirkin BR and Ewing LL (1989) Kinetic studies on the development of the adult population of Leydig cells in testes of the pubertal rat. Endocrinology 124: 762–770.

Hess KR, Zhang W, Baggerly KA, Stivers DN and Coombes KR (2001) Microarrays: handling the deluge of data and extracting reliable information. Trends Biotechn 19: 463–468.

Höög C (1991) Isolation of a large number of novel mammalian genes by a differential cDNA library screening strategy. Nucl Acids Res 19: 6123–6127.

Ivell R, Pera I, Ellerbrock K, Beiglböck A, Gebhardt K, Osterhoff C, Kirchhoff C. (1998) The dog as a model system to study epididymal gene expression. J. Reprod. Fertil. Suppl. 53: 33–45.

Jin H, Cheng X, Diatchenko L, Siebert PD and Huang CC (1997) Differential screening of a subtracted cDNA library: a method to search for genes preferentially expressed in multiple tissues. Biotechniques 23: 1084–1086.

Kirchhoff C, Osterhoff C, Habben I and Ivell R (1990) Cloning and analysis of mRNAs specifically expressed in the human epididymis. Int J Androl 13: 155–167

Kleene KC, Distel RJ and Hecht NB (1983) cDNA clones encoding cytoplasmic polyA+ RNAs which first appear at detectable levels in haploid phases of spermatogenesis. Dev Biol 98: 455–464.

Liang P and Pardee AB (1992) Differential display of eukaryotic messenger RNA by means of the polymerase chain reaction. Science 257: 967–971.

Maniatis T, Fritsch EF and Sambrook J (1982) Molecular Cloning: A laboratory Manual. Coldspring Harbor Laboratory Press, New York.

Naaby-Hansen S, Flickinger CJ and Herr JC (1997) Two-dimensional gel electrophoresic analysis of vectorially labeled surface proteins of human spermatozoa. Biol Reprod 56: 771–787.

Ozaki K, Kuroki T, Hayashi S and Nakamura Y (1996) Isolation of three testis-specific genes (TSA303, TSA806, TSA903) by a differential display method. Genomics 36: 316–319.

Pusch W, Balvers M and Ivell R (1996a) Molecular cloning and expression of the relaxin-like factor from the mouse testis. Endocrinology 137: 3009–3013.

Pusch W, Balvers M, Hunt, N and Ivell R (1996) A novel endozepine–like peptide (ELP) is exclusively expressed in male germ cells. Mol Cell Endocrinol 127: 69–80

Schröter S, Derr P, Conradt HS, Nimitz M, Hale G and Kirchhoff C (1999) Male-specific modification of human CD52. J Biol Chem 247: 29862–29873.

Spiess AN, Ivell R (2002) A highly efficient method for long-chain cDNA synthesis using trehalose and betaine. Anal. Biochem. (in press).

Thomas KH, Wilkie TM, Tomashefsky P, Bellvé AR and Simon MI (1989) Differential gene expression during mouse spermatogenesis. Biol Reprod 41: 729–739.

Willison K, Dudley K, Potter J (1986) Molecular cloning and sequence analysis of a haploid expressed gene encoding t-complex polypeptide I. Cell 44: 727–738.

Yang Z, Wreford NG and de Kretser D (1990) A quantitative study of spermatozoa in the developing rat testis. Biol Reprod 43: 629–635.

9 Spermatogonial Stem Cell Development

D.G. de Rooij, L.B. Creemers, K. den Ouden, F. Izadyar

9.1 The Origin of Spermatogonial Stem Cells and Their Precursors

Spermatogonial stem cells originate from primordial germ cells (PGCs) that derive from epiblast cells (embryonal ectoderm) (Lawson and Pederson 1992). During fetal development the PGCs proliferate and migrate to the genital ridges, where they become enclosed in the seminiferous cords formed by Sertoli cell precursors. Once in the seminiferous cords, the cells are called gonocytes which are morphologically different from the PGCs (Clermont and Perey 1957; Huckins and Clermont 1968;

Sapsford 1962). Gonocytes proliferate for a while and then become quiescent. In mice and rats, gonocytes start spermatogenesis shortly after birth and give rise to spermatogonial stem cells as well as the first A1 spermatogonia (review de Rooij 1998).

PGCs are single cells that in culture can form colonies of cells which morphologically resemble undifferentiated embryonic stem cells (ES cells; Resnick et al. 1992). On feeder layers, these cells can be maintained for a long period of time and can give rise to embryoid bodies and to various cell types in monolayer culture. Primordial-germ-cell-derived ES cells can contribute to chimaeras when injected into host blastocysts (Resnick et al. 1992). Hence, PGCs are stem cells that still have the capacity to differentiate in various directions.

The next cell type in the spermatogenic cell lineage, the gonocytes, can only be cultured in the presence of Sertoli cells (van Dissel-Emiliani et al. 1993), while PGCs can be co-cultured with other types of somatic cells. Furthermore, it has been shown that already in gonocytes cytokinesis is not completed, leading to the formation of intercellular bridges between daughter cells (Zamboni and Merchant 1973). As described below, in the adult testis intercellular bridge formation designates the cells for differentiation and consequently many gonocytes may already be destined to differentiate along the spermatogenic lineage. From these data it can be concluded that most likely in the spermatogenic lineage the multipotentiality of the stem cells is lost at the transition from PGCs to gonocytes.

9.2 Spermatogenesis in the Adult

Spermatogenesis starts with a series of mitotic divisions carried out by spermatogonia. The last mitotic division renders spermatocytes that go through S phase, then pass through the lengthy prophase of the first meiotic division and subsequently carry out the two meiotic divisions to give rise to haploid spermatids. Initially, spermatids have a round shape but then elongate to become spermatozoa that leave the seminiferous tubules through the tubule lumen (review Russell et al. 1990).

The spermatogenic process can continue during the entire lifespan of a male. This is made possible by the stem cells that are at the basis of spermatogenic process. Spermatogonial stem cells are both able to self-renew and to give rise to differentiating daughter spermatogonia. This dual capacity of stem cells ensures the long-lasting ability of the testes to produce spermatozoa. Spermatogonia are situated on the basal membrane of the seminiferous tubules. Various subsequent types of spermatogonia can be distinguished that will be discussed below. As in this respect there is a considerable difference between primate- and non-primate mammals, non-primates will be discussed first and the situation in primates will be described separately.

9.3 Spermatogonial Stem Cells in Non-Primate Mammals

Spermatogonial stem cells are single cells that are located on the basal membrane of the seminiferous tubules and are called A-single (A_s) spermatogonia (de Rooij 1973; de Rooij and Russell 2000; Huckins 1971c; Oakberg 1971). These cells either divide into two new single cells or into a pair of daughter cells (A_{pr} spermatogonia) that do not complete cytokinesis and stay connected by an intercellular bridge (Fawcett et al. 1959; Weber and Russell 1987). Subsequently, in all further divisions, starting with the pair, cytokinesis will also be incomplete, leading to the formation of increasingly large syncytia of germ cells. Hence, all differentiating progeny of a spermatogonial stem cell will stay connected by intercellular bridges, which is a unique characteristic compared to other renewing tissues. As A_{pr} spermatogonia are morphologically similar to A_s spermatogonia, the intercellular bridge is the first visible sign of the entry into the differentiation pathway.

9.4 Symmetrical or Asymmetrical Stem Cell Divisions?

It is not known yet whether the divisions of spermatogonial stem cells are symmetrical or not (de Rooij and Russell 2000). When there is just one pool of stem cells in which these cells have an about 50% chance of giving rise to two stem cell daughters or to a pair of cells that will differentiate, i.e. Apr spermatogonia, divisions are symmetrical. In contrast, there could be a situation in which there are two kinds of stem cells. One that will always divide into single daughter cells and one that has an increased chance to give rise to Apr spermatogonia. This implies asymmetrical divisions of the first kind of spermatogonial stem cells, one of the daughter cells remaining in the stem cell line, the other being predestined to become Apr spermatogonia after one or more divisions.

Several reports have addressed this question. Based on cell kinetic data in the rat Huckins (1971a) concluded that there are spermatogonial stem cells with a very long cell cycle that preferentially self-renew and stem cells that cycle more quickly and preferentially divide into Apr spermatogonia. However, in a similar, but more extensive study in the Chinese hamster this conclusion could not be confirmed (Lok et al. 1984). Nevertheless, recent data obtained by culturing bovine spermatogonia do point to a heterogeneity in the stem cell population. As discussed in more detail below, two types of self-sustaining spermatogonial colonies were formed during long-term culture of bovine spermatogonia. One type of colonies was composed of single cells with a uniform appearance and one also contained chains of cells. Presumably, in one type there are only spermatogonial stem cells that do not differentiate and in the other at least some of the daughter cells enter the differentiation pathway.

9.5 Differentiating Pathway

The first cells in the spermatogenic lineage destined to develop into spermatozoa are the A_{pr} spermatogonia (Fig. 1). These A_{pr} spermatogonia divide further to form chains of 4, 8, up to occasionally 32 so-called A-aligned (A_{al}) spermatogonia. The A_{al} spermatogonia can go through a differentiation step and become so-called A1 spermatogonia. This differentiation step involves slight morphological changes (Chiarini Garcia and Russell 2001) and brings about a change in cell cycle characteristics of the spermatogonia (Huckins 1971b; Huckins 1971d; Lok and de Rooij 1983a; Lok et al. 1983). While A_s, A_{pr} and A_{al} spermatogonia cycle more or less at random, the A1 spermatogonia and following generations of spermatogonia proliferate with a fixed cell cycle time, which, for example in the mouse, is about 30 h (Monesi 1962). In most non-primate mammals there are six divisions following the formation of A1 spermatogonia, the last one of which giving rise to spermatocytes. In total, in rodents there are about 10 spermatogonial

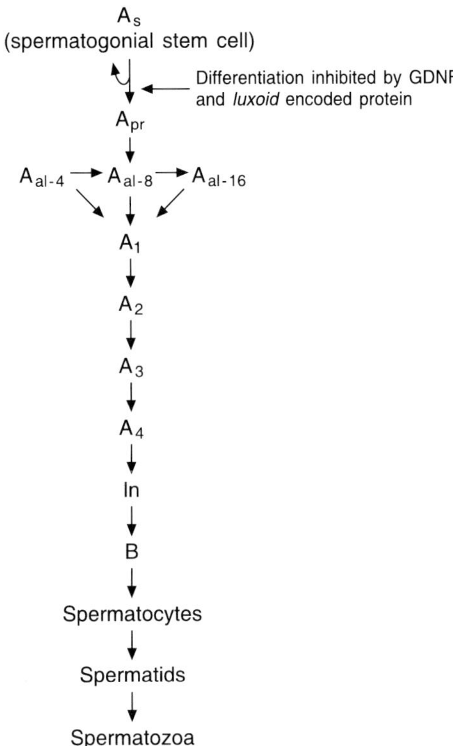

Fig. 1. Scheme of the subsequent types of cells in the spermatogenic lineage in the mouse and rat and the supposed way spermatogonial multiplication and stem cell renewal takes place. Molecules involved in the regulation of stem cell renewal and differentiation are also indicated

divisions between the spermatogonial stem cells and the formation of spermatocytes (de Rooij and Russell 2000).

The proliferative activity of spermatogonial stem cells depends on the stages of the cycle of the seminiferous epithelium. In between stages X and III the stem cells divide two to three times and in the other part of the epithelial cycle they are largely quiescent (Lok and de Rooij 1983b; Tegelenbosch and de Rooij 1993). During the whole cycle of the seminiferous epithelium, the numbers of stem cells and A_{pr} spermatogonia remain about the same (Lok et al. 1982; Tegelenbosch and de Rooij 1993). The A_s spermatogonia either divide into A_{pr} or into new A_s spermatogonia. The A_{pr} spermatogonia divide further to become A_{al} spermatogonia and consequently during the period of active proliferation, more and more A_{al} spermatogonia are formed. Once every epithelial cycle, the A_{al} spermatogonia differentiate into A1 spermatogonia that start the series of (mostly 6) divisions to become spermatocytes.

9.6 Morphological Identification and Cell Cycle Characteristics of Spermatogonial Stem Cells

Spermatogonial stem cells can be recognized morphologically using whole mounts of seminiferous tubules (Clermont and Bustos-Obregon 1968). These whole mounts enable one to study the topography of the spermatogonia lying on the basal membrane and to distinguish singles, pairs and chains of these cells. Hence, differential cell counts of stem cells, A_{pr} and A_{al} spermatogonia can be carried out. Furthermore, a method was developed to perform autoradiography on these whole mounts (Huckins and Kopriwa 1969). Using ^{3}H-thymidine and the labeled mitoses technique, it was found that spermatogonial stem cells have a relatively long cell cycle time of at least 56 h in the rat (Huckins 1971b) and 90 h in the Chinese hamster (Lok et al. 1983). These cell cycle times resemble those of A_{pr} and A_{al} spermatogonia but are longer than in subsequent types of spermatogonia (Huckins 1971d; Lok and de Rooij 1983a).

9.7 Purification of Spermatogonial Stem Cells

In the adult mouse testis, there are about 35,000 stem cells which is only 0.03% of all germ cells (Tegelenbosch and de Rooij 1993).Various techniques have been developed to purify the total population of A spermatogonia, achieving a purity varying between 85 to 98% (Bellve et al. 1977; Dirami et al. 1999; Morena et al. 1996). Unfortunately, in the mouse only about 3% of the A spermatogonia are stem cells (Tegelenbosch and de Rooij 1993) and it will not likely be much different in other animals. Hence, although a 100-fold enrichment of stem cells can be achieved by purifying A spermatogonia, the purity is still very low. To further increase the purity, a method has been developed to isolate spermatogonia from vitamin A deficient rats (van Pelt et al. 1996). In vitamin A deficient rats and mice spermatogenesis is arrested at the differentiation step of A_{al} into A1 spermatogonia and the testes of these animals only contain A_s, A_{pr} and A_{al} spermatogonia (van Pelt and de Rooij 1990). Starting from testes of vitamin A deficient animals, a cell population containing about 10% stem cells can be obtained (Tegelenbosch and de Rooij 1993; van Pelt et al. 1996).

Certain biochemical markers have been used to enrich spermatogonial stem cells (Shinohara and Brinster 2000; Shinohara et al. 1999). Using anti-β1- and anti-α6-integrin and negatively selecting for the c-kit receptor, which is not present on spermatogonial stem cells (Schrans-Stassen et al. 1999), a 40-fold enrichment of spermatogonial stem cells from testicular germ cells could be accomplished (Shinohara et al. 1999).

Taken together, the purification of spermatogonial stem cells has not yet reached further than a purity of about 10% at most. More specific membrane markers for these cells will have to be found to achieve further progress in this field.

9.8 Spermatogonial Cultures

Attempts have been made to culture pure populations of stem cells in the absence of serum or a feeder layer. Unfortunately, these attempts have been less successful in that few cells survive 1 week of culture (Dirami et al. 1999; Creemers et al., to be published. However, in a long-term culture of a mixed germ cell suspension, in the presence of serum and on a feeder layer, some spermatogonial stem cells did survive and were able to repopulate a recipient mouse testis after transplantation (Nagano et al. 1998). Long-term survival (25 days) and proliferation of mouse spermatogonia cultured with Sertoli cells and in the presence of serum has also been achieved (van der Wee et al. 2001). Recently, a bovine spermatogonia/Sertoli cell co-culture system was developed allowing survival, proliferation and differentiation up to spermatids, during at least 4 months (Izadyar et al. 2002). In these cultures, 2 types of spermatogonial colo-

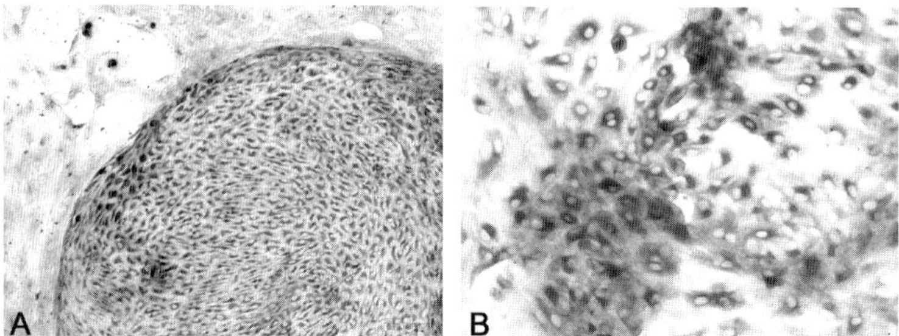

Fig. 2A, B. Colonies observed after long-term culture of bovine spermatogonia. The bovine spermatogonia are immunohistochemically stained for binding of the spermatogonia-specific lectin DBA. **A** Round colony consisting of single, uniform cells. **B** Radial colony in which besides single cells, groups of cells are also seen

nies were formed, one consisting of only single stem cells and a mixed type in which besides stem cells also pairs and chains of cells were formed (Fig. 2). Intriguingly, these data again suggest the existence of two types of stem cells, one prone to differentiate and one only capable of self-renewal without the proper stimulus.

9.9 Spermatogonial Stem Cell Transplantation

The presence of spermatogonial stem cells and/or their functionality can be examined by the spermatogonial transplantation technique developed by Brinster and coworkers (Brinster and Avarbock 1994; Brinster and Zimmermann 1994). In this technique, germ cells of one mouse are transplanted into the testes of a recipient mouse, the endogenous spermatogenesis of which is depleted by treatment of the mice with the alkylating agent busulfan. Also mice carrying the *Wv/Wv* mutation can be used as recipients, the testes of which do not contain germ cells. Recently, a reliable and effective method to kill the endogenous spermatogonial stem cells in the recipient mice has been developed using fractionated X-irradiation (local testicular doses of 1.5 and 12 Gy, 24 h apart). This protocol causes more than 95% depletion (Creemers et al. 2002). After transplantation the donor stem cells repopulate the seminiferous epithelium of the recipient mice. Interestingly, also rat spermatogonial stem cells are able to repopulate the mouse testis and produce normal rat spermatogenesis in the mouse (Clouthier et al. 1996; Russell and Brinster 1996). However, stem cells from other species transplanted into mouse testes either produce defective spermatogenesis (hamster; Ogawa et al. 1999) or initiate repopulation by spermatogonia only (rabbit and dog, Dobrinski et al. 1999; bull, Izadyar et al. 2001). In the latter species, pairs and chains of A spermatogonia are formed, indicating that donor spermatogonial stem cells do produce differentiating A_{pr} spermatogonia but these cells fail to develop further.

9.10 Regulation of Stem Cell Renewal and Differentiation

Like all other renewing tissues, the seminiferous epithelium is able to react to (stem) cell loss by the initiation of enhanced stem cell renewal in order to replace the lost stem cells. The potential of recovery of spermatogonial stem cells has been studied extensively at the cellular level by studying the reaction of the seminiferous epithelium to irradiation. It was found that after a high dose of irradiation, surviving spermatogonial stem cells almost only self-renew during at least their first 6 divisions, leading to a rapid recovery of stem cell numbers in those areas where one or more stem cells survived (van Beek et al. 1990). Nothing is known yet about the triggers involved in preventing stem cell differentiation or enhancing self-renewal in such a situation.

In several renewing tissues, stem cells were found to occupy specific areas. For example in the intestine, stem cells reside near the bottom of the crypts (Potten 1998) and stem cells in the bone marrow are also supposed to occupy specific niches (Schofield 1983). Until recently, in the seminiferous epithelium no such niches were found for spermatogonial stem cells. Now it has become clear that most spermatogonial stem cells are present in those areas of seminiferous tubules that border on interstitial tissue (Chiarini Garcia et al. 2001). Apparently, the interstitial tissue affects stem cell behavior in such a way that differentiation is less likely to occur when the stem cells lie close to it. Possibly, this is caused by the high testosterone levels present in these areas. Interestingly, high testosterone levels have been found to prevent the differentiation of A_{al} spermatogonia into A1 spermatogonia (Shetty et al. 2001; Shuttlesworth et al. 2000; Tohda et al. 2001). Possibly, testosterone also has a role in regulating stem cell behavior. However, one has to keep in mind that germ cells do not possess androgen receptors so that testosterone can only indirectly affect spermatogonia via peritubular myoid cells or (more likely) Sertoli cells that both express this receptor.

The ratio between self-renewal and differentiation of spermatogonial stem cells being under the control of regulatory mechanisms, the question arises which molecular pathways are involved in these mechanisms. Recent data indicate that glial cell line derived neurotrophic factor (GDNF) is involved. Normally, GDNF is secreted by Sertoli cells (Trupp et al. 1995) while a subset of spermatogonia express the receptors for this growth factor, Ret and GFR-alpha1 (Meng et al. 2000). Ectopic expression of GDNF in spermatogonia induces the formation of large clusters of single type A spermatogonia, while normal spermatogenesis is suppressed. Moreover, in mice overexpressing GDNF in spermatogonia, germ cell tumors that resemble human seminoma, are formed at about 1 year of age (Meng et al. 2001). GDNF deficient mice die during the first postnatal day (Pichel et al. 1996) whereas heterozygotes survive. In heterozygotes spermatogenesis deteriorates with age as germ cells become depleted (Meng et al. 2000). It was concluded that GDNF has a role in the regulation of self-renewal and differentiation of spermatogonial stem cells (Fig. 1). Too high levels of GDNF inhibit stem cell differentiation and cause an accumulation of stem cells and low levels stimulate differentiation and cause stem cell depletion.

Another interesting recent finding in this field is that in the classical spontaneous mouse mutant *luxoid*, adult males exhibit a progressive loss of spermatogonial stem cells (Braun et al. 2001). Apparently, the as yet unknown gene(s) involved in this mutation also has a role in the regulation of spermatogonial stem cell renewal and differentiation (Fig. 1).

9.11 Spermatogonial Stem Cells in Primates

Spermatogonial multiplication and stem cell renewal in primates has been described in much less detail than in rodents. As in rodents, in primates there are A and B spermatogonia but the composition of the type A spermatogonial population is complicated. Primate A spermatogonia have been subdivided into A_{pale} and A_{dark} spermatogonia according to their staining with hematoxylin (Clermont 1966a). The A_{pale}

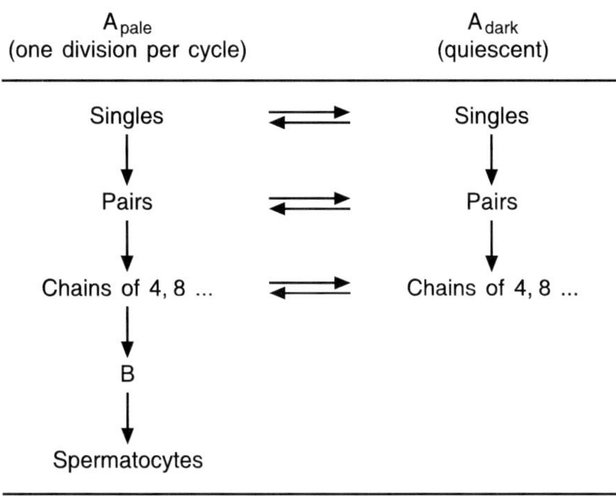

Fig. 3. Hypothetical scheme of spermatogonial multiplication and stem cell renewal in primates

spermatogonia divide once every cycle of the seminiferous epithelium. In the human, this means that they divide only once every 16 days (Clermont 1966b; Heller and Clermont 1963). A_{dark} spermatogonia in the normal epithelium are quiescent cells and are supposed to be reserve (stem) cells (Fig. 3).

An important question is whether A_{pale} and A_{dark} spermatogonia are stem cells. To answer this question, an obvious approach is to look at the topographical arrangement of these spermatogonia on the basal membrane. In the normal seminiferous epithelium the density of A_{pale} and A_{dark} spermatogonia is relatively high. Therefore the clones are too close together to decide whether or not A_{pale} and A_{dark} spermatogonia consist of clones of 1 or 2^n cells comparable to spermatogonia in non-primate mammals. However, such a clonal arrangement can be observed for both A_{pale} and A_{dark} spermatogonia during repopulation after irradiation when spermatogonial density is much lower (van Alphen et al. 1988a). In that situation singles, pairs and chains of A_{pale} and A_{dark} spermatogonia can be observed in tubule whole mounts. As it seems unlikely that the spermatogonial compartment would be principally different between primates and non-primate mammals likely only the single cells among the A_{pale} and A_{dark} spermatogonia have stem cell properties (de Rooij 1983; van Alphen et al. 1988a).

It has generally been assumed that A_{dark} spermatogonia are reserve (stem) cells. The first real evidence for such a reserve function came from a study in rhesus monkeys. Shortly after irradiation, it was found that the number of A_{pale} spermatogonia gradually decreased to a minimum at about day 9 after irradiation, while there was no change in the number of A_{dark} spermatogonia (van Alphen et al. 1988b). This pattern can be explained by the different proliferative activity of these cells. After irradiation, lethally damaged cells go into apoptosis when they divide and consequently the proliferating A_{pale} die and the quiescent A_{dark} survive. However, after longer intervals than 9 days, the A_{dark} spermatogonia also decreased in number concomitantly with a transient rise in the number of A_{pale}. Finally, both cell types dropped to very low numbers. The transient nature of the increase in A_{pale} after more than 9 days after irradiation can be explained by assuming that after the initial decline in A_{pale} numbers, the A_{dark} spermatogonia are activated. The activation first causes the A_{dark} to acquire the A_{pale} appearance and accompanying proliferative activity. Then having become A_{pale}, they tried to divide but due to the lethal radiation damage, acquired during the time when they were still A_{dark}, proper division fails and the cells enter apoptosis.

In conclusion, the A_{pale} and A_{dark} spermatogonia in primates are topographically arranged in singles, pairs and chains of spermatogonia (Fig. 3). Unless spermatogonial renewal and multiplication in primates is totally different from that in non-primate mammals only the singles among them are stem cells and are comparable to the A_s in non-primates. Only the A_{pale} spermatogonia are able to proliferate and do so once every epithelial cycle. From this it can be deduced that the formation of a chain of 8 from a differentiating stem cell will take 3 cycles, i.e. 48 days in the human. The A_{dark} spermatogonia are quiescent and only are activated after cell loss. When these cells are activated they become A_{pale} spermatogonia first and then start to proliferate. During repopulation by surviving stem cells new A_{dark} spermatogonia are set aside again (van Alphen et al. 1988a). Comparing primate to non-primate spermatogenesis it is clear that there is much less proliferative activity of the stem cells in the primate seminiferous epithelium, even by the active stem cells, the A_{pale}. A quiescent stem cell compartment, the A_{dark}, is missing in non-primate mammals. The low proliferative activity of spermatogonial stem cells in primates seems advantageous since this lowers the chance of errors in DNA duplication during S phase. The less stem cells divide the better (Lajtha 1979).

9.12 Perspectives in Spermatogonial Stem Cell Research

While until recently the emphasis of spermatogonial research was more on the regulation of the A_s, A_{pr} and A_{al} spermatogonia as a group, now specific data on the molecular regulation of spermatogonial stem cell behavior are rapidly emerging. GDNF and its receptors, and the gene involved in the *luxoid* mutation, seem directly involved in the regulation of stem cell renewal and differentiation. Furthermore, testosterone clearly has an indirect role and may even be responsible for the intriguing fact that spermatogonial stem cells are preferably present in those areas of seminiferous tubules that border on interstitial tissue. These findings together with the possibility to do functional tests for stem cell potential by way of the spermatogonial stem cell transplantation technique, as well as the progress that is recently made in developing culture techniques open this field for new approaches to establish the regulatory mechanisms that govern spermatogonial stem cell renewal and differentiation.

Acknowledgements. This work is supported by grants from the Netherlands Technological Foundation (STW) and the National Institutes of Health (USA).

References

Bellve AR, Cavicchia JC, Millette CF, O'Brien DA, Bhatnagar YM, Dym M (1977) Spermatogenic cells of the prepuberal mouse. Isolation and morphological characterization. J Cell Biol 74:68–85

Braun RE, Nadler JJ, Buaas FW, Morris JL, Connolly CM (2001) Genetic analysis of the male germ line. In Abstract book XVIth Testis Workshop Regulatory mechanisms of testicular cell differentiation, Newport Beach:28

Brinster RL, Avarbock MR (1994) Germline transmission of donor haplotype following spermatogonial transplantation. Proc Natl Acad Sci USA 91:11303–11307

Brinster RL, Zimmermann JW (1994) Spermatogenesis following male germ-cell transplantation. Proc Natl Acad Sci USA 91:11298–11302

Chiarini Garcia H, Russell LD (2001) High-resolution light microscopic characterization of mouse spermatogonia. Biol Reprod 65:1170–1178

Chiarini Garcia H, Hornick JR, Griswold MD, Russell LD (2001) Distribution of type A spermatogonia in the mouse is not random. Biol Reprod 65:1179–1185

Clermont Y (1966a) Spermatogenesis in man. A study of the spermatogonial population. Fertil Steril 17:705–721

Clermont Y (1966b) Renewal of spermatogonia in man. Am J Anat 118:509–524

Clermont Y, Perey B (1957) Quantitative study of the cell population of the seminiferous tubules of immature rats. Am J Anat 100:241–268

Clermont Y, Bustos-Obregon E (1968) Re-examination of spermatogonial renewal in the rat by means of seminiferous tubules mounted "in toto". Am J Anat 122:237–247

Clouthier DE, Avarbock MR, Maika SD, Hammer RE, Brinster RL (1996) Rat spermatogenesis in mouse testis. Nature 381:418–421

Creemers LB, den Ouden K, Meng X, Sariola H, van Pelt AMM, Izadyar F, Santoro M, de Rooij DG (2002) transplantation of germ cells from GDNF overexpressing mice to host testes depleted from endogenous spermatogenesis by fractionated irradiation. Submitted.

de Rooij DG (1973) Spermatogonial stem cell renewal in the mouse. I. Normal situation. Cell Tissue Kinet 6:281–287

de Rooij DG (1983) Proliferation and differentiation of undifferentiated spermatogonia in the mammalian testis. In: Potten CS (ed) Stem cells. Their identification and characterization. Churchill Livingstone, Edinburgh:89–117

de Rooij DG (1998) Stem cells in the testis. Int J Exp Pathol 79:67–80

de Rooij DG, Russell LD (2000) All you wanted to know about spermatogonia but were afraid to ask. J Androl 21:776–798

Dirami G, Ravindranath N, Pursel V, Dym M (1999) Effects of stem cell factor and granulocyte macrophage-colony stimulating factor on survival of porcine type A spermatogonia cultured in KSOM. Biol Reprod 61:225–230

Dobrinski I, Avarbock MR, Brinster RL (1999) Transplantation of germ cells from rabbits and dogs into mouse testes. Biol Reprod 61:1331–1339

Fawcett DW, Ito S, Slautterback DL (1959) The occurrence of intercellular bridges in groups of cells exhibiting synchronous differentiation. J Biophys Biochem Cytol 5:453–460

Heller CG, Clermont Y (1963) Spermatogenesis in man: an estimate of its duration. Science 140:184–185

Huckins C (1971a) The spermatogonial stem cell population in adult rats. 3. Evidence for a long-cycling population. Cell Tissue Kinet 4:335–349

Huckins C (1971b) The spermatogonial stem cell population in adult rats. II. A radioautographic analysis of their cell cycle properties. Cell Tissue Kinet 4:313–334

Huckins C (1971c) The spermatogonial stem cell population in adult rats. I. Their morphology, proliferation and maturation. Anat. Rec. 169:533–557

Huckins C (1971d) Cell cycle properties of differentiating spermatogonia in adult Sprague- Dawley rats. Cell Tissue Kinet 4:139–154

Huckins C, Clermont Y (1968) Evolution of gonocytes in the rat testis during late embryonic and early post-natal life. Arch Anat Histol Embryol 51:341–354

Huckins C, Kopriwa BM (1969) A technique for the radioautography of germ cells in whole mounts of seminiferous tubules. J Histochem Cytochem 17:848–851

Izadyar F, Creemers LB, den Ouden K, de Rooij DG (2001) Culture and transplantation of bovine spermatogonial stem cells. In: Robaire B, Chemes HE, Morales CR (eds) Andrology in the 21st century. Medimond, Englewood:149–155

Izadyar F, den Ouden K, Creemers LB, Posthuma G, de Rooij DG (2002) Proliferation and differentiation of type A spermatogonia during long term culture. Submitted

Lajtha LG (1979) Stem cell concepts. Differentiation 14:23–34

Lawson KA, Pederson RA (1992) Clonal analysis of cell fate during gastrulation and early neurulation in the mouse. In Ciba Foundation Symposium 165. Post implantation development in the mouse. John Whiley & Sons, New York:3–26

Lok D, de Rooij DG (1983a) Spermatogonial multiplication in the Chinese hamster. I. Cell cycle properties and synchronization of differentiating spermatogonia. Cell Tissue Kinet 16:7–18

Lok D, de Rooij DG (1983b) Spermatogonial multiplication in the Chinese hamster. III. Labelling indices of undifferentiated spermatogonia throughout the cycle of the seminiferous epithelium. Cell Tissue Kinet 16:31–40

Lok D, Weenk D, de Rooij DG (1982) Morphology, proliferation, and differentiation of undifferentiated spermatogonia in the Chinese hamster and the ram. Anat Rec 203:83–99

Lok D, Jansen MT, de Rooij DG (1983) Spermatogonial multiplication in the Chinese hamster. II. Cell cycle properties of undifferentiated spermatogonia. Cell Tissue Kinet 16:19–29

Lok D, Jansen MT, de Rooij DG (1984) Spermatogonial multiplication in the Chinese hamster. IV. Search for long cycling stem cells. Cell Tissue Kinet 17:135–143

Meng X, Lindahl M, Hyvonen ME, Parvinen M, de Rooij DG, Hess MW, Raatikainen-Ahokas A, Sainio K, Rauvala H, Lakso M, Pichel JG, Westphal H, Saarma M, Sariola H (2000) Regulation of cell fate decision of undifferentiated spermatogonia by GDNF. Science 287:1489–1493

Meng XJ, de Rooij DG, Westerdahl K, Saarma M, Sariola H (2001) Promotion of seminomatous tumors by targeted overexpression of glial cell line-derived neurotrophic factor in mouse testis. Cancer Res 61:3267–3271

Monesi V (1962) Autoradiographic study of DNA synthesis and the cell cycle in spermatogonia and spermatocytes of mouse testis using tritiated thymidine. J Cell Biol 14:1–18

Morena AR, Boitani C, Pesce M, De Felici M, Stefanini M (1996) Isolation of highly purified type A spermatogonia from prepubertal rat testis. J Androl 17:708–717

Nagano M, Avarbock MR, Leonida EB, Brinster CJ, Brinster RL (1998) Culture of mouse spermatogonial stem cells. Tissue Cell 30:389–397

Oakberg EF (1971) Spermatogonial stem-cell renewal in the mouse. Anat Rec 169:515–531

Ogawa T, Dobrinski I, Avarbock MR, Brinster RL (1999) Xenogeneic spermatogenesis following transplantation of hamster germ cells to mouse testes. Biol Reprod 60:515–521

Pichel JG, Shen L, Sheng HZ, Granholm AC, Drago J, Grinberg A, Lee EJ, Huang SP, Saarma M, Hoffer BJ, Sariola H, Westphal H (1996) Defects in enteric innervation and kidney development in mice lacking GDNF. Nature 382:73–76

Potten CS (1998) Stem cells in gastrointestinal epithelium: numbers, characteristics and death. Philos Trans R Soc Lond B Biol Sci 353:821–830

Resnick JL, Bixler LS, Cheng L, Donovan PJ (1992) Longterm proliferation of mouse primordial germ cells in culture. Nature 359:550–551

Russell LD, Brinster RL (1996) Ultrastructural observations of spermatogenesis following transplantation of rat testis cells into mouse seminiferous tubules. J Androl 17:615–627

Russell LD, Ettlin RA, Hikim APS, Clegg ED (1990) Histological and histopathological evaluation of the testis. Cache River Press, Clearwater, Fl. USA

Sapsford CS (1962) Changes in the cells of the sex cords and the seminiferous tubules during development of the testis of the rat and the mouse. Austr J Zool 10:178–192

Schofield R (1983) The stem cell system. Biomed Pharmacother 37:375–380

Schrans-Stassen BHGJ, van de Kant HJG, de Rooij DG, van Pelt AMM (1999) Differential expression of c-kit in mouse undifferentiated and differentiating type A spermatogonia. Endocrinology 140:5894–5900

Shetty G, Wilson G, Huhtaniemi I, Boettger-Tong H, Meistrich ML (2001) Testosterone inhibits spermatogonial differentiation in juvenile spermatogonial depletion mice. Endocrinology 142:2789–2795

Shinohara T, Brinster RL (2000) Enrichment and transplantation of spermatogonial stem cells. Int J Androl 23 Suppl. 2:89–91

Shinohara T, Avarbock MR, Brinster RL (1999) beta(1)- and alpha(6)-integrin are surface markers on mouse spermatogonial stem cells. Proc Natl Acad Sci USA 96:5504–5509

Shuttlesworth GA, de Rooij DG, Huhtaniemi I, Reissmann T, Russell LD, Shetty G, Wilson G, Meistrich ML (2000) Enhancement of A spermatogonial proliferation and differentiation in irradiated rats by GnRH antagonist administration. Endocrinology 141:37–49

Tegelenbosch RA, de Rooij DG (1993) A quantitative study of spermatogonial multiplication and stem cell renewal in the C3H/101 F1 hybrid mouse. Mutat Res 290:193–200

Tohda A, Matsumiya K, Tadokoro Y, Yomogida K, Miyagawa Y, Dohmae K, Okuyama A, Nishimune Y (2001) Testosterone suppresses spermatogenesis in juvenile spermatogonial depletion (jsd) mice. Biol Reprod 65:532–537

Trupp M, Ryden M, Jornvall H, Funakoshi H, Timmusk T, Arenas E, Ibanez CF (1995) Peripheral expression and biological activities of GDNF, a new neurotrophic factor for avian and mammalian peripheral neurons. J Cell Biol 130:137–148

van Alphen MMA, van de Kant HJG, de Rooij DG (1988a) Repopulation of the seminiferous epithelium of the rhesus monkey after X irradiation. Radiat Res 113:487–500

van Alphen MMA, van de Kant HJG, de Rooij DG (1988b) Depletion of the spermatogonia from the seminiferous epithelium of the rhesus monkey after X irradiation. Radiat Res 113:473–486

van Beek MEAB, Meistrich ML, de Rooij DG (1990) Probability of self-renewing divisions of spermatogonial stem cells in colonies, formed after fission neutron irradiation. Cell Tissue Kinet 23:1–16

van der Wee KS, Johnson EW, Dirami G, Dym M, Hofmann MC (2001) Immunomagnetic isolation and long-term culture of mouse type A spermatogonia. J Androl 22:696–704

van Dissel-Emiliani FM, de Boer-Brouwer M, Spek ER, van der Donk JA, de Rooij DG (1993) Survival and proliferation of rat gonocytes in vitro. Cell Tissue Res 273:141–147 van Pelt AMM, de Rooij DG (1990) The origin of the synchronization of the seminiferous epithelium in vitamin A-deficient rats after vitamin A replacement. Biol Reprod 42:677–682

van Pelt AMM, Morena AR, van Dissel-Emiliani FMF, Boitani C, Gaemers IC, de Rooij DG, Stefanini M (1996) Isolation of the synchronized A spermatogonia from adult vitamin A- deficient rat testes. Biol Reprod 55:439–444

Weber JE, Russell LD (1987) A study of intercellular bridges during spermatogenesis in the rat. Am J Anat 180:1–24

Zamboni L, Merchant H (1973) The fine morphology of mouse primordial germ cells in extragonadal locations. Am J Anat 137:299–335

10 Multimeric Coactivator Complexes for Steroid/Nuclear Receptors

L.P. Freedman

Nuclear receptors regulate transcription in direct response to their cognate hormonal ligands. Ligand-binding leads to the dissociation of corepressors and the recruitment of coactivators. Many of these factors, acting in large complexes, have emerged as chromatin remodelers through intrinsic histone-modifying activities or through other novel functions. In addition, other ligand-recruited complexes appear to act more directly on the transcriptional apparatus, suggesting that transcriptional regulation by nuclear receptors may involve a process of both chromatin alterations and direct recruitment of key initiation components at regulated promoters.

10.1 Introduction

Nuclear receptors comprise a very large family of ligand-inducible transcription factors. Like other eukaryotic factors that regulate transcription, nuclear receptors bind selectively to DNA, primarily as di-

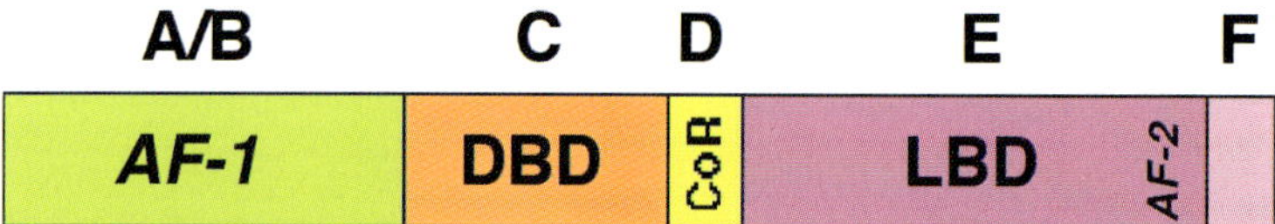

Fig. 1. Functional domains of nuclear receptors. A/B and F domains vary in size and primary sequence among the superfamily. *CoR* refers to corepressor binding site present in some nuclear receptors. *AF-1* and *AF-2* refer to two distinct activation functions (see text)

mers through two characteristic zinc finger modules and a dimerization region that directs self-interaction or hetero-partnering. Moreover, they possess identifiable transactivation functions (AF's) which can independently confer activation potential to heterologous DNA-binding domains. Transactivation is mediated by both constitutive and inducible AF's (AF-1 and AF-2, respectively; Fig. 1), the latter of which is conferred by its integral location within the ligand-binding domain (LBD).

The ligands for nuclear receptors include steroids, retinoids, vitamin D, thyroid hormone, prostanoids, and cholesterol metabolites, such as oxysterols and bile acids. Their combined effects are vast, influencing virtually every fundamental biological process, from development and homeostasis, to proliferation and differentiation. For example, retinoids and vitamin D3 are potent growth inhibitors and inducers of differentiation, particularly of cells of immune and hematopoietic lineages. In addition, PPARγ ligands have a remarkable effect on the induction of adipocyte differentiation. The elucidation of the mechanisms by which nuclear receptors regulate cellular processes will require both the identification of key target genes, as well as a detailed accounting of the molecular events that are initiated by the highly specific and tight interactions that occur between ligand and receptor leading to transactivation. This review will focus on the latter question, with an emphasis on how ligand-binding facilitates the recruitment of receptor-associated protein complexes that in turn affect transcription initiation at regulated promoters.

10.2 Histone-Modifying Cofactors

Cellular DNA is packaged into chromatin, a repeating array of a protein:DNA complex of which the minimal and recently crystallographically defined unit is the nucleosome, consisting of a histone octamer enveloped by 146 bp of DNA [1]. Yeast genetics correlated the acetylation state of the N-terminal tails of histones to gene expression and provided the first evidence for how chromatin might be regulated to control transcription [2, 3]. From these and other studies it was postulated that hyperacetylation of histones promoted an "open" transcriptionally active state, and hypoacetylation a "closed" transcriptionally repressed state. A large number of nuclear receptor transcriptional "coactivators" and "corepressors" have been recently isolated . identified genetically and biochemically in yeast, mammalian cells, and from extracts in vitro that harbor histone -acetylase (HAT) or -deacetylase (HDAC) activities and have been suggested to act by remodeling chromatin. When deacetylase inhibitors such as Trichostatin-A or butyrate have been utilized in cells or in vitro, chromatin derepression and increased transcription have been observed [4–6]. One family of related proteins are collectively termed the p160 coactivators. They are represented by SRC-1/NCoA-1, TIF2/GRIP1/NCoA-2, and pCIP/ACTR/AIB1. LBD's were used as baits since an essential ligand-dependent transactivation function mapped to the C-terminus of this domain (AF-2; Fig. 1). A second, ligand-independent activation function (AF-1) resides within the N-terminus of many but not all nuclear receptors. Besides sequence homology, p160 proteins share an ability to stimulate ligand-dependent transactivation by a rather large number of nuclear receptors in transient overexpression experiments. A distinctive structural feature of the p160 coactivators is the presence of multiple LXXLL signature motifs (also called LXDs, NR boxes, or NIDs), which comprise determinants for direct interactions with the nuclear receptor AF-2.

Although the amino acid context surrounding the LXXLL motif appears to influence selectivity of interaction, it is unclear at this point what, if anything, influences the specificity of nuclear receptor/p160 binding. Several recent LBD crystal structures have established that upon ligand binding, the an α-helix containing the AF-2 core (helix 12) undergoes a major reorientation in the context of the overall LBD

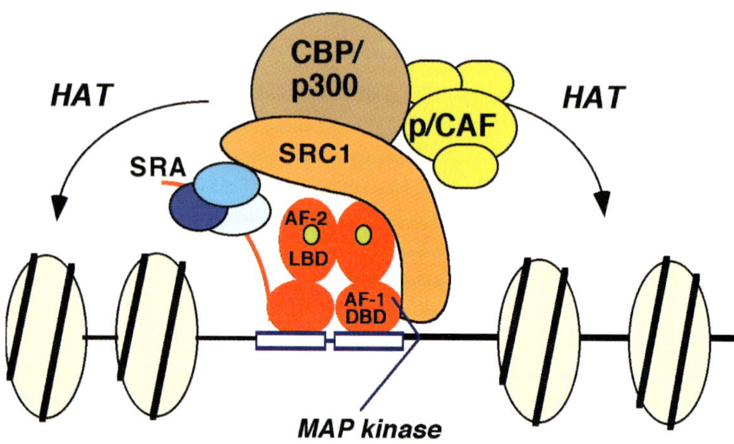

Fig. 2. p160 Coactivators such as SRC-1 anchor a complex comprising CBP/p300 and p/CAF and other factors to nuclear receptors through ligand-dependent AF-2 interactions and, in some cases, MAP kinase-inducible phosphorylation sites in the AF-1. The net effect of these interactions would be to provide HAT activity, resulting in a remodelling of chromatin

structure, forming part of a "charged clamp" that accommodates p160 coactivators within a hydrophobic cleft of the LBD; this occurs through direct contacts with the LXXLL motif (reviewed in ref. 7 and references therein). Remarkably, estrogen antagonists such as tamoxifen and raloxifene appear to alter the position of the AF-2 core such that helix 12 itself occupies the hydrophobic cleft in the LBD, thereby precluding coactivator binding [8, 9]. In fact, several experiments preceding these crystal structure analyses indicated that a key mechanistic effect of hormonal antagonists is to inhibit p160 interaction with the LBD, further supporting the biological relevance of coactivators in nuclear receptor function.

Insight into a potential mechanism of p160 coactivation came with the finding that SRC-1 is capable of interacting with the C-terminus of CBP/p300 and together they can coactivate synergistically [10]. In addition, CBP/p300 itself interacts directly with nuclear receptors in a ligand-dependent manner, again through the AF-2 domain [11, 12]. Thus one can imagine a growing HAT-containing, chromatin-remodelling complex comprising CBP, p160, and p/CAF recruited to nuclear receptors in response to hormone-binding (Fig. 2). While some of these individual proteins have been observed to exert significant transcriptional effects when overexpressed or limited in cells (particularly CBP [12] and SRC-1/NCoA-1 [13–15]) or biochemically in vitro (p300) [16], it is becoming increasingly clear that they are associated with other polypeptides, many of which were originally identified as direct nuclear receptor interacting proteins. For coactivators, these include pCAF/GCN5, p/CIP/AIB1/ACTR, and GRIP-1/TIF2. As mentioned above, these proteins have been reported to contain intrinsic HAT activity. Moreover, p/CAF, the mammalian homologue of the prototypical yeast HAT, GCN5, is part of a 20 or so subunit complex containing TAFs and TAF-like proteins [17]; it interacts with both CBP and some p160 coactivators, as well as directly with nuclear receptors [18, 19]. The corepressors N-CoR and SMRT have been found as part of large complexes containing Sin3-A and -B, rpd3/HDAC-1 and -2, the latter possessing histone deacetylase activities [20–22]. Thus, these proteins may act in concert to modify histone tails and could thereby destabilize or stabilize chromatin. Since these same proteins have also been found to directly modify several transactivators, including p53 [23] and GATA-1 [24], as well as components of the general transcription machinery [25], their direct role in chromatin remodeling remains uncertain and could be limited to modulation of enhancer binding affinity in a local chromatin context. Nevertheless, these complexes may be related to the yeast GCN5-containing SAGA, ADA, NuA3 and NuA4 HAT complexes, which have been demonstrated to direct chromatin-dependent transcription by select activators in vitro in response to acetyl-CoA [26].

10.2.1 Contacts with RNA Polymerase II: The DRIP Coactivator Complex

A recently discovered multi-subunit complex that binds to vitamin D receptor (VDR) [32, 33] thyroid hormone receptor (TR) [34] and, most likely, many other members of the steroid/nuclear receptor family, points to the ultimate generality of transactivation. This complex, alternatively called TRAP or DRIP, is recruited to the nuclear receptor LBD

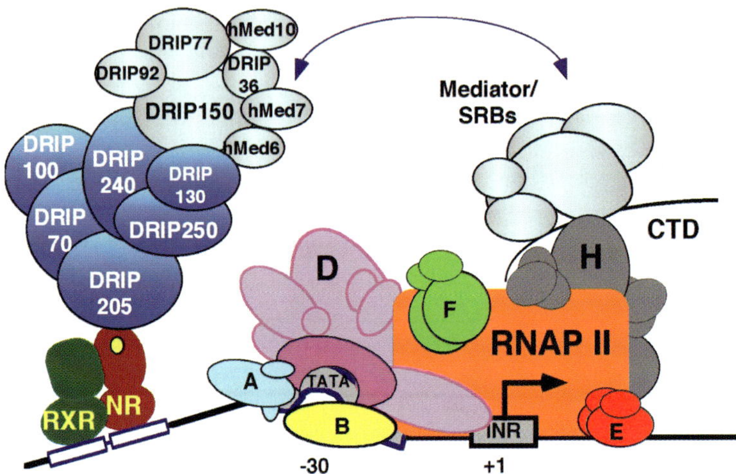

Fig. 3. A coactivator complex comprising DRIP/TRAP/ARC and Mediator/SRB subunits is recruited to nuclear receptors in a ligand-dependent manner through a single subunit, DRIP205 (TRAP220). Shown here is a DNA-bound nuclear receptor/RXR heterodimer. Mediator/SRB subunits that are shared between the nuclear receptor/DRIP/TRAP/ARC complex (*silver*) and RNA Pol II suggests that coactivation by the DRIP/TRAP/ARC complex can occur, at least in part, through recruitment or stabilization of RNA Pol II. Chromatin remodeling coactivators such as the p160/CBP/PCAF complex might bind directly to steroid/nuclear receptors or perhaps through ligand-recruited coactivators such as the DRIP/ARC/TRAP complex, opening up the chromatin to then allow the DRIP/ARC/TRAP complex to act directly on the preinitiation complex, potentially through shared SRB/Mediator subunits

AF-2 in response to ligand-binding most likely through a single subunit (DRIP205/TRAP220). However, this single subunit anchors an additional 13–15 proteins comprising the DRIP/TRAP complex, thereby conferring hormone-dependent recruitment of what appears to be a preformed complex. The generality of this complex stems from the surprising observation that other activators unrelated to steroid/nuclear receptors, such as VP16, p65 subunit of NFkB, and SREBP-1a, recruit this complex (called ARC) [35] and that many of the DRIP/TRAP/ARC subunits are present in three similar, if not identical, SRB-associated complexes, NAT, SMCC, and mammalian SRB/Mediator, targeted by adenovirus E1A [36–38]. Most importantly, these related complexes are required for transcriptional activation by these same activators as demonstrated utilizing purified components in in vitro transcription assays.

At least seven DRIP/ARC/TRAP subunits are homologous to proteins described as components of Mediator, a complex originally found both to be required for transcription in a yeast model system in vitro and, together with SRBs, able to associate with yeast RNA polymerase II (Pol II) through its large subunit's Carboxyl Terminal repeat Domain (CTD) [39]. A similar complex was subsequently found to associate with a mammalian Pol II CTD [40]. Yeast genetics of homologous subunits and preliminary biochemical observations allude to its potential role in recruitment of or contact with the Pol II machinery at the core promoter (Fig. 3). It is also plausible, however, that DRIP/ARC/TRAP may intrinsically contain or interact with as yet undefined chromatin remodeling activities. The direct biochemical roles of this multi-protein coactivator complex as well as those of the structurally-related cofactor, CRSP [41], recently identified as required for Sp1 transactivation from naked DNA templates, await further characterization.

10.3 Conclusions and Perspectives

Steroid and nuclear receptors have evolved to directly regulate the transcription of many genes in order to accommodate intricate metazoan developmental and differentiation programs in rapid response to environmental cues. In recent years, molecular genetics and biochemistry have identified many intermediary components, co-activators and co-repressors, involved in both ligand-dependent and ligand-independent signaling by these receptors as well as their direct target genes. How the DRIP/ARC/TRAP complex interfaces with the p160/CBP/pCAF system, for example, is an intriguing question. Given the current accepted role for the p160/CBP/pCAF complex functioning at the level of chromatin remodelling through intrinsic HAT activity, and the fact that DRIP/ARC/TRAP does not contain a HAT [33], one could envision a two-step process for these two complexes. In this model, chromatin remodeling coactivators bound directly to steroid/nuclear receptors could open up the chromatin to then allow the DRIP/ARC/TRAP complex to act directly on the preinitiation complex, potentially through shared SRB/Mediator subunits.

A further understanding of which intermediary factors are involved in the transcriptional control of particular target genes will require direct examination of endogenous loci and transgenes in a chromatin context within cells in concert with the continued development of highly integrated transcription systems that respond to multiple activators in a chromatin context in vitro. These types of experiments will allow for further identification of novel cofactors and the dissection and elucidation of the direct biochemical functions of particular chromatin modifying, remodeling, and general cofactors in coordinating the action of nuclear receptors and other classes of activators and repressors at complex promoters.

References

1. Luger K, Mäder AW, Richmond RK, Sargent DF and Richmond TJ. (1997) Crystal structure of the nucleosome core particle at 2.8 Å resolution. Nature 389, 251–260.
2. Kayne PS, Kim U, Han M, Mullen JR, Yoshizaki F and Grunstein M (1988) Extremely conserved histone H4 N terminus is dispensable for growth but essential for repressing the silent mating loci in yeast. Cell 55, 27-39.
3. Megee PC, Morgan BA, Miltman BA and Smith MM (1990) Genetic analysis of histone H4: essential role of lysines subject to reversible acetylation. Science 247, 841–845.
4. Sheridan PL, Mayall TP, Verdin E and Jones KA (1997) Histone acetyltransferases regulate HIV-1 enhancer activity in vitro. Genes Dev. 11, 3327–3340.
5. Côté J, Peterson CL and Workman JL (1998) Perturbation of nucleosome core structure by the SWI/SNF complex persists after its detachment, enhancing subsequent transcription factor binding. Proc. Natl. Acad. Sci. USA 95, 4947–4952.
6. Nightingale KP, Wellinger RE, Sogo JM and Becker PB (1998) Histone acetylation facilitates RNA polymerase II transcription of the Drosophila hsp26 gene in chromatin. EMBO J 17, 2865–2876.
7. Xu, L., Glass, C. K., and Rosenfeld, M. G. (1999) Coactivator and corepressor complexes in nuclear receptor function. Curr. Opin. Genet. Dev. 9, 140–147.

8. Brzozowski, A. M., Pike, A. C., Dauter, Z., Hubbard, R. E., Bonn, T., Engstrom, O., Ohman, L., Greene, G. L., Gustafsson, J. A., and Carlquist, M. (1997) Molecular basis of agonism and antagonism in the estrogen receptor. Nature 389, 753–758.

9. Shiau, A. K., Barstad, D., Loria, P. M., Cheng, L., Kushner, P. J., Agard, D. A., and Greene, G. L. (1998) The structural basis of estrogen receptor/coactivator recognition and the antagonism of this interation by tamoxifen. Cell 95, 927–937.

10. Yao, T. P., Ku, G., Zhou, N., Scully, R., and Livingston, D. M. (1996) The nuclear hormone receptor coactivator SRC-1 is a specific target of p300. Proc. Natl. Acad. Sci. USA 93, 10626–10631.

11. Chakravarti, D., Lamorte, V.J., Nelson, M.C., Nakajima, T., Schulman, I.G., Juguilon, H., Montminy, M., and Evans, R.M. (1996) Role of CBP/p300 in nuclear receptor signalling. Nature 383, 99–103.

12. Kamei Y, Xu L, Heinzel T, Torchia J, Kurokawa R, Gloss B, Lin SC, Heyman RA, Rose DW, Glass CK and Rosenfeld MG (1996) A CBP integrator complex mediates transcriptional activation and AP-1 inhibition by nuclear receptors. Cell 85, 403–14.

13. Spencer TE, Jenster G, Burcin MM, Allis CD, Zhou J, Mizzen CA, McKenna NJ, Onate SA, Tsai SY, Tsai M-J and O'Malley BW (1997) Steroid receptor coactivator-1 is a histone acetyltransferase. Nature 389, 194–198.

14. Onate SA, Tsai SY, Tsai MJ and O'Malley BW (1995) Sequence and characterization of a co-activator for the steroid hormone receptor superfamily. Science 270, 1354–1357.

15. McInerney EM, Rose DW, Flynn SE, Westin S, Mullen T-M, Krones A, Inostroza J, Torcia J, Assa-Munt N, Milburn MV, Glass CK and Rosenfeld MG (1998) Determinants of coactivator LXXLL motif specificity in nuclear receptor transcriptional activation. Genes Dev. 12, 3357–3368.

16. Kraus WL and Kadonaga JT (1998) p300 and estrogen receptor cooperatively activate transcription via differential enhancement of initiation and reinitiation. Genes Dev. 12, 331–342.

17. Ogryzko, V.V., Kotani, T., Zhang, X.L., Schlitz, R.L., Howard, T., Yang, X.J., Howard, B.H., Qin, J., and Nakatani, Y. (1998) The transcriptional coactivators p300 and CBP are histone acetyltransferases. Cell 94, 35-44.

18. Chen H, Lin RJ, Schiltz RL, Chakravarti D, Nash A, Nagy L, Privalsky ML, Nakatani Y and Evans RM (1997) Nuclear receptor coactivator ACTR is a novel histone acetyltransferase and forms a multimeric activation complex with P/CAF and CBP/p300. Cell 90, 569–580.

19. Blanco, J. C. G., Minucci, S., Lu, J. M., Yang, X. J., Walker, K. K., Chen, H. W., Evans, R.M., Nakatani, Y., and Ozato, K. (1998) The histone acetylase PCAF is a nuclear receptor coactivator. Genes Dev. 12, 1638–1651.

20. Nagy L, Kao HY, Chakravarti D, Lin RJ, Hassig CA, Ayer DE, Schreiber SL and Evans RM (1997) Nuclear receptor repression mediated by a complex containing SMRT, mSin3 A, and histone deacetylase. Cell 89, 373–380.
21. Heinzel T, Lavinsky RM, Mullen T-M, Söderström M, Laherty CD, Torchia J, Yang W-M, Brard G, Ngo SD, Davie JR, Seto E, Eisenman RN, Rose DW, Glass CK and Rosenfeld MG (1997) A complex containing N-CoR, mSin3 and histone deacetylase mediates transcriptional repression. Nature 387, 43–48.
22. Alland L, Muhle R, Hou HJ, Potes J, Chin L, Screiber-Agus N and DePinho RA (1997) Role for N-CoR and histone deacetylase in Sin3-mediated transcriptional repression. Nature 387, 49–55.
23. Gu W and Roeder RG (1997) Activation of p53 sequence-specific DNA binding by acetylation of the p53 C-terminal domain. Cell 90, 595–606.
24. Hung HL, Lau J, Kim AY, Weiss MJ and Blobel GA (1999) CREB-binding protein acetylates hematopoietic transcription factor GATA-1 at important sites. Mol Cell Biol 19, 3496–505.
25. Imhof A, Yang XJ, Ogryzko VV, Nakatani Y, Wolffe AP and Ge H (1997) Acetylation of general transcription factors by histone acetyltransferases. Curr Biol 7, 689–692.
26. Utley RT, Ikeda K, Grant PA, Côté J, Steger DJ, Eberharter A, John S and Workman JL (1998) Transcriptional activators direct histone acetyltransferase complexes to nucleosomes. Nature 394, 498–502.
27. Lanz, R. B., McKenna, N. J., Onate, S. A., Albrecht, U., Wong, J., Tsai, S. Y., Tsai, M.-J., and O'Malley, B. W. (1999) A steroid receptor coactivator, SRA, functions as an RNA and is present in an SRC-1 complex. Cell 97, 17–27.
28. Tremblay, A., Tremblay, G. B., Labrie, F., and Giguere, V. (1999) Ligand-independent recruitment of SRC-1 to estrogen receptor β through phosphorylation of activation function AF-1. Mol. Cell 3, 513–520.
29. Hammer, G. D., Krylova, I., Zhang, Y., Darimont, B. D., Simpson, K., Weigel, N. L., and Ingraham, H. A. (1999) Phosphorylation of the nuclear receptor SF-1 modulates cofactor recruitment: integration of hormone signalling in reproduction and stress. Mol. Cell 3, 521–528.
30. Hu, E., Kim, J. B., Sarraf, P., and Spiegelman, B. M. (1996) Inhibition of adipogenesis through MAP kinase-mediated phosphorylation of PPAR-γ. Science 274, 2100–2103.
31. Shao, D., Rangwala, S. M., Bailey, S. T., Krakow, S. L., Reginato, M. J., and Lazar, M. A. (1998) Interdomain communication regulating ligand binding by PPAR-γ. Nature 396, 377–380.
32. Rachez C, Suldan Z, Ward J, Chang CP, Burakov D, Erdjument-Bromage H, Tempst P and Freedman LP (1998) A novel protein complex that inter-

acts with the vitamin D3 receptor in a ligand-dependent manner and enhances VDR transactivation in a cell-free system. Genes Dev. 12, 1787–1800.

33. Rachez C, Lemon BD, Suldan Z, Bromleigh V, Gamble M, Näär AM, Erdjument-Bromage H, Tempst P and Freedman LP (1999) Ligand-dependent transcription activation by nuclear receptors requires the DRIP complex. Nature 398, 824–828.

34. Fondell JD, Ge H and Roeder RG (1996) Ligand induction of a transcriptionally active thyroid hormone receptor coactivator complex. Proc. Natl. Acad. Sci. USA 93, 8329–8333.

35. Näär AM, Beaurang PA, Zhou S, Abrahams A, Solomon W and Tjian R (1999) Composite coactivator ARC mediates chromatin-directed transcriptional activation. Nature 398, 828–832.

36. Sun X, Zhang Y, Cho H, Rickert P, Lees E, Lane W and Reinberg D (1998) NAT, a human complex containing Srb polypeptides that functions as a negative regulator of activated transcription. Mol Cell 2, 213–222.

37. Ito M, Yuan C-X, Malik S, Gu W, Fondell JD, Yamamura S, Fu Z-Y, Zhang X, Qin J and Roeder RG (1999) Identity between TRAP and SMCC complexes indicates novel pathways for the function of nuclear receptors and diverse mammalian activators. Mol. Cell 3, 361–370.

38. Boyer TG, Martin MED, Lees E, Ricciardi RP and Berk AJ (1999) Mammalian Srb/Mediator complex is targeted by adenovirus E1 A protein. Nature 399, 276–279.

39. Kim Y-J, Bjorkland S, Li Y, Sayre MH and Kornberg RD (1994) A multiprotein mediator of transcriptional activation and its interaction with the C-terminal repeat domain of RNA Polymerase II. Cell 77, 599–608.

40. Jiang YW, Veschambre P, Erdjument-Bromage H, Tempst P, Conaway JW, Conaway RC and Kornberg RD (1998) Mammalian mediator of transcriptional regulation and its possible role as an end-point of signal transduction pathways. Proc. Natl. Acad. Sci. U S A 95, 8538–8543.

41. Ryu S, Zhou S, Ladurner AG and Tjian R (1999) The transcriptional cofactor complex CRSP is required for activity of the enhancer-binding protein Sp1. Nature 397, 446–450.

42. Wong, J, Patterton, D, Imhof, A, Guschin, D, Shi, Y-B, and Wolf, AP (1998) Distinct requirements for chromatin assembly in transcriptional repression by thyroid hormone receptor and histone deacetylase. EMBO J 17, 520–534.

43. Hittelman, A.D., Burakov, D., Iñiguez-Lluhí, J.A., Freedman, L.P., and Garabedian, M.J. (1999) Differential regulation of glucocorticoid receptor transcriptional activation via AF-1-associated proteins. EMBO J., in press.

11 DAX1 and SF1 Mutations Provide Insight into Sexual Differentiation

G. Ozisik, J.C. Achermann, J.J. Meeks, J.L. Jameson

11.1 Introduction

Testis determination in humans requires a series of developmental "switches" that direct differentiation of the Sertoli and Leydig cells from progenitor cells in the bipotential gonad (or genital ridge). These biological events are initiated by a transient wave of *SRY* (sex-related gene on the Y chromosome) expression that alters the fate of cells in the indifferent gonad to give rise to Sertoli instead of ovarian granulosa cells (Albrecht and Eicher 2001). Once Sertoli cells form, they coalesce into tubules and support germ cell development. Sertoli cells also produce factors such as MIS (Müllerian Inhibiting Substance, also known as Anti-Müllerian Hormone, AMH) and inhibin that affect testis development and the function of neighboring cells. MIS causes the regression of Müllerian structures precluding formation of the fallopian tubes, uterus, and upper segment of the vagina. Leydig cells secrete testosterone, which is necessary for development of the male external genitalia and development of the Wolffian structures including the epididymides, vasa

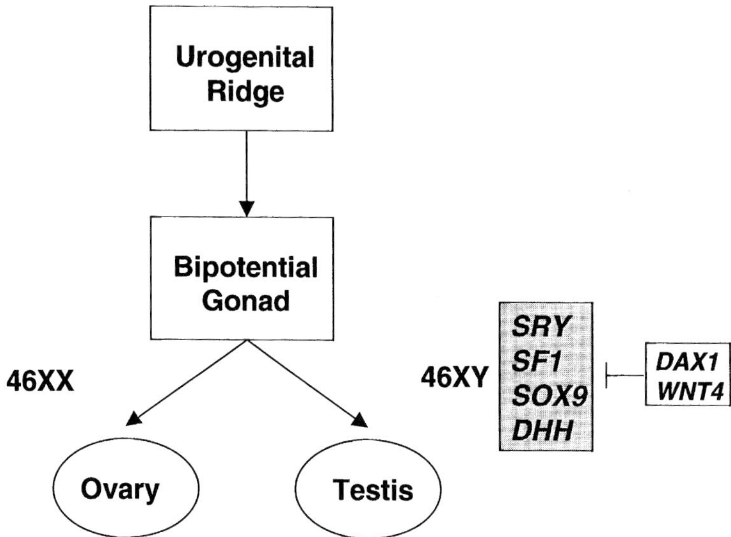

Fig. 1. Gonadogenesis during embryonic and fetal development. The genes required for testis differentiation are *shaded*

deferentia, and seminal vesicles. Together, the combined activities of these hormones produce a normal male internal and external reproductive tract (MacLaughlin et al. 2001).

The genetic cascade that leads to testis determination is under tight transcriptional control (Fig. 1). The Y-chromosomal gene, *SRY*, is a pivotal switch for male-specific differentiation. The mechanism of *SRY* action remains unclear but as a member of the HMG (high mobility group)-box family of transcription factors, it is likely that SRY interacts with other transcription factors to selectively alter the expression of target genes. The expression of *SOX9* (SRY-related HMG-box gene 9) is strikingly upregulated in the developing male gonad and turned off in the female gonad. Targeted expression of *Sox9* is sufficient to initiate testis formation and mutations that disrupt *SOX9* impair testis development, indicating that it is a key gene in testis determination (Kwok et al. 1995; Vidal et al. 2001). Whether *SOX9* is a downstream target of SRY or is regulated independently of SRY is currently unknown. SOX9 binds to a specific site in the *MIS* promoter, and synergizes with SF1 (steroidogenic factor-1) to regulate tissue-specific expression of *MIS*. SF1 is required for adrenal and gonadal development (both testis and ovary) and appears to function in conjunction with other transcription factors to regulate a large group of adrenal and gonadal genes (see below). The expression pattern of SF1 parallels that of another orphan nuclear receptor, DAX1 (dosage sensitive sex-reversal, adrenal hypoplasia congenita on the X chromosome, gene 1), in the gonad. In contrast to *Sox9*, *Dax1* is downregulated in the developing testis but not in the ovary, suggesting that *Dax1* is not required for testis formation. Overexpression of *Dax1* inhibits *Sry*-mediated testis determination, suggesting that Dax1 may act as an "anti-testis" factor (Swain and Lovell-Badge 1999). The exquisite sensitivity of the male sex-determining pathways to gene dosage is apparent in humans, as duplication of *DAX1* results in 46XY sex-reversal (see below). In addition to those mentioned above, many other genes (e.g., *WT1*, *GATA4*, *WNT4*, *DHH*, and *FATE*) are also involved in gonadal differentiation and development as well as final positioning of the gonads (i.e., *INSL3*, *HOXA10*, *HOXA11*). This chapter will focus on *DAX1* and *SF1*, which act at various stages of sex-determination, but also contribute to the development and function of the entire reproductive endocrine network.

11.2 X-Linked Adrenal Hypoplasia Congenita and *DAX1*

Identification of single gene defects that influence the reproductive axis at multiple levels (including the hypothalamus, pituitary, and gonad) have provided useful insight into the processes that regulate the development of the GnRH neurons, gonadotropes, adrenals, and testes. Adrenal hypoplasia congenita (AHC) is a rare disorder characterized by adrenal insufficiency and hypogonadotropic hypogonadism (HHG). Mutations or deletions of *DAX1* (*AHC, NR0B1*) cause the X-linked cytomegalic form of AHC (MIM 300200) (Muscatelli et al. 1994). Typically, boys with this condition present with severe primary adrenal failure in infancy or childhood. HHG becomes apparent at puberty and infertility results from gonadotropin deficiency in combination with a primary defect in spermatogenesis (Habiby et al. 1996; Seminara et al. 1999).

Duplication of the region of Xp containing the *DAX1* locus is associated with dosage-sensitive XY sex-reversal in humans (Bardoni et al.

1994). Overexpression of its murine homologue (*Ahch, Dax1*) causes sex-reversal in male mice in the background of a weakened *Sry* allele (temporally delayed) (Swain et al. 1998). Thus, overactivity as well as underactivity of DAX1 can have important effects on gonadal development and reproductive function, demonstrating the importance of gene dosage effects in the development of this biological system.

11.2.1 Structure, Expression and Function of DAX1

DAX1 is a 470-aa transcription factor with a carboxy-terminal region that resembles the ligand binding domain (LBD) of other nuclear receptors. However, the amino-terminal half of this protein consists of a unique repeat structure (Fig. 2) that contains several LXXLL-like motifs implicated in protein-protein interactions (Zhang et al. 2000). The carboxyterminus of DAX1 confers potent transcriptional silencing activity (Ito et al. 1997; Lalli et al. 1997). The crystal structure of DAX1 is yet to be resolved and it is unclear whether there is a ligand for DAX1 that might alter is structure and transcriptional activity.

Dax1/DAX1 is expressed in the developing urogenital ridge from E10.5 in mice and 33 dpo in humans. Subsequently, *Dax1/DAX1* is expressed in the primordial adrenal gland, the fetal adrenal gland, and in all layers of the adult adrenal cortex (Guo et al. 1995; Hanley et al. 2000; Ikeda et al. 1996). Expression is also detected in the developing diencephalon (E11.5) and pituitary gonadotropes (E14.5) in mice, and in the hypothalamus and pituitary in humans, consistent with a role in gonadotropin production (Ikeda et al. 2001). The differentiating mouse

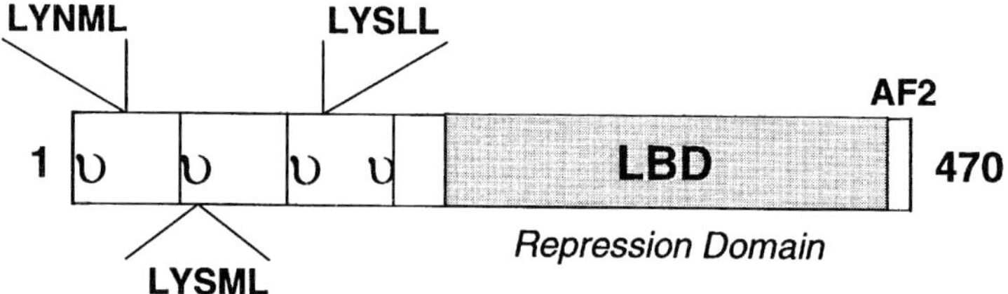

Fig. 2. Schematic representation of DAX1. Putative LBD and AF2 domain are located in the carboxy-terminal half of the protein, which possesses potent repressor activity. The 66–67 amino acid repeat motifs consist of three LXXLL-like core sequences that have been implicated in protein–protein interactions

gonad expresses *Dax1* until E12, after which there is a rapid decline in the testis, but continued expression in the ovary (Ikeda et al. 1996). This sexually dimorphic pattern of expression initially suggested that *Dax1* may play a role in sex determination, either as an ovarian determining gene or as a repressor of testicular development. However, targeted disruption of *Dax1* does not interfere with ovarian development (Yu et al. 1998). *Dax1* is also expressed in the mature testis (Guo et al. 1995; Tamai et al. 1996), where it appears to play a role in differentiation and function of Sertoli and Leydig cells (Jeffs et al. 2001b; Yu et al. 1998).

Although loss of DAX1 function is associated with adrenal failure and HHG in humans, the majority of functional data suggest that DAX1 is a repressor of gene transcription. This repression is mediated by direct protein-protein interactions or corepressor recruitment (Altincicek et al. 2000; Crawford et al. 1998; Zhang et al. 2000). Additional evidence suggests that DAX1 may also act at the level of post-transcriptional processing by binding to and shuttling mRNA from the nucleus (Lalli et al. 2000).

Activation of gene transcription by nuclear receptors is often dependent on the recruitment of coactivators via a region containing an LXXLL core consensus sequence (Heery et al. 1997). Although these leucine-rich motifs, referred to as NR boxes, are characteristic for most AF2 coactivators, DAX1 and its closest relative SHP (short heterodimer partner) have been shown to utilize such motifs for their repressor interactions with ligand-activated estrogen receptors (Johansson et al. 2000; Zhang et al. 2000). Consistent with these observations, the interaction between DAX1 and SF1 is mediated by the amino-terminal half of the DAX1 protein, suggesting that at least one NR box is involved in this interface (Ito et al. 1997).

11.2.2 Human *DAX1* (*NR0B1*) Mutations

Over 80 different mutations in *DAX1* have been described (Phelan and McCabe 2001), most of which are nonsense or frameshift mutations that cause premature truncation of the protein. Deletion of as few as the last nine amino acids of DAX1, which constitute a putative AF2 domain, is associated with a severe clinical phenotype (Nakae et al. 1996). Relatively few missense mutations have been reported in *DAX1*. These

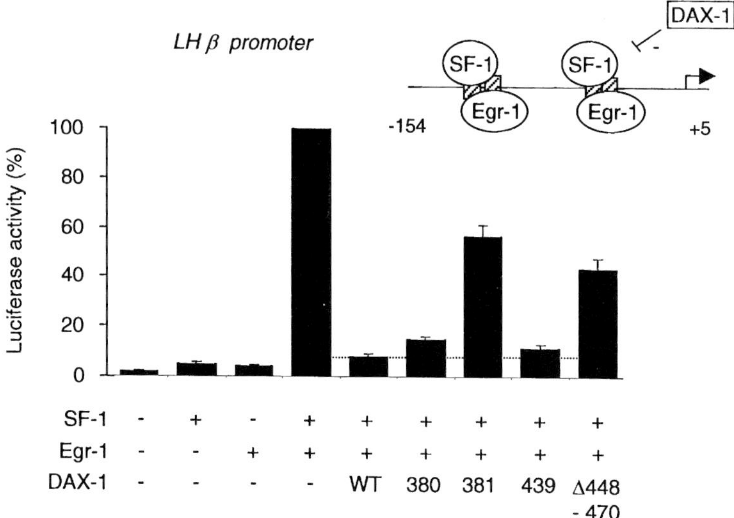

Fig. 3. Synergistic activation of the LHβ gene promoter by SF1/Egr1 is repressed by wild-type DAX1. The missense mutation L381H, and carboxy-terminal deletion mutant (amino acids 448–470) show a loss of repression, and represent naturally occurring missense and truncation mutants, respectively. The Y380D and I439S mutations have partial loss of function. The latter mutations were found in two males who presented with a mild form of AHC in adulthood. (Reproduced with permission from Mantovani et al. 2002)

mutations appear to cluster within certain regions of the carboxy-terminus of DAX1, and may provide insight into potentially important domains for DAX1 function (Zhang et al. 1998; Achermann et al. 2001).

Current data suggest that there is little correlation between the type or position of *DAX1* mutation and age at presentation or diagnosis (Reutens et al. 1999). "Early" or "late" clinical presentation can be a feature even within the same family in which two or more siblings harbor the same *DAX1* mutation. Further, most DAX1 mutations result in similar loss of transcriptional repression in functional assays, despite somewhat variable clinical presentations. These observations suggest that modifier genes or environmental factors account for much of variability in the AHC clinical presentation. Rarely, patients have been identified with relatively mild DAX1 missense mutations that result in partial loss of transcriptional repression (Fig. 3). It is of interest that these individuals first presented in adulthood with evidence of mild adrenal failure or partial HHG (Mantovani et al. 2002; Tabarin et al. 2000). However, the absence of *DAX1* mutations in a relatively large group of patients with familial and sporadic forms of HHG and delayed puberty indicates that mutations are unlikely in such patients without associated adrenal failure (Achermann et al. 1999a). Thus, while most *DAX1* mutations result in total or near-total loss of function, mutations with some residual function may rarely be associated with milder or delayed AHC phenotypes.

The association of HHG with X-linked AHC is well established and appears to reflect a functional role for DAX1 at the level of the pituitary (gonadotrope cells) as well as the hypothalamus (ventromedial hypothalamic effect on GnRH production) (Habiby et al. 1996; Seminara et al. 1999; Tabarin et al. 2000). Pulsatile gonadotropin-releasing hormone (GnRH) has been used in an attempt to induce puberty or fertility in patients with *DAX1* mutations but it is unusual to normalize gonadotropin levels with this approach. Gonadotropins have been used in an attempt to stimulate testosterone production and induce spermatogenesis. Though testosterone levels are often normalized, the limited data available suggest that it is difficult to induce spermatogenesis using exogenous gonadotropins in patients with *DAX1* mutations (Mantovani et al. 2002; Seminara et al. 1999; Tabarin et al. 2000). This finding may reflect a direct effect of DAX1 on Sertoli cell development and spermatogenesis (Jeffs et al. 2001a).

11.2.3 Targeted Mutagenesis of *Dax1* (*Ahch*)

Targeted mutagenesis of *Dax1* was used to produce a murine model of X-linked AHC and to study the role of *Dax1* in development (Yu et al. 1998). A "Cre-loxP" targeting strategy was necessary as Dax1 seems to be essential for embryonic stem (ES) cell survival and because mutations in *Dax1* cause infertility in males (ES cells are XY-derived). No gross abnormalities in adrenal function were detected in knockout mice, although there is a delay in adrenal X-zone regression that may mimic the human adrenal phenotype to some extent (Babu et al. 2002). The most striking effect of the mutation was seen in the testis. Male *Dax1*

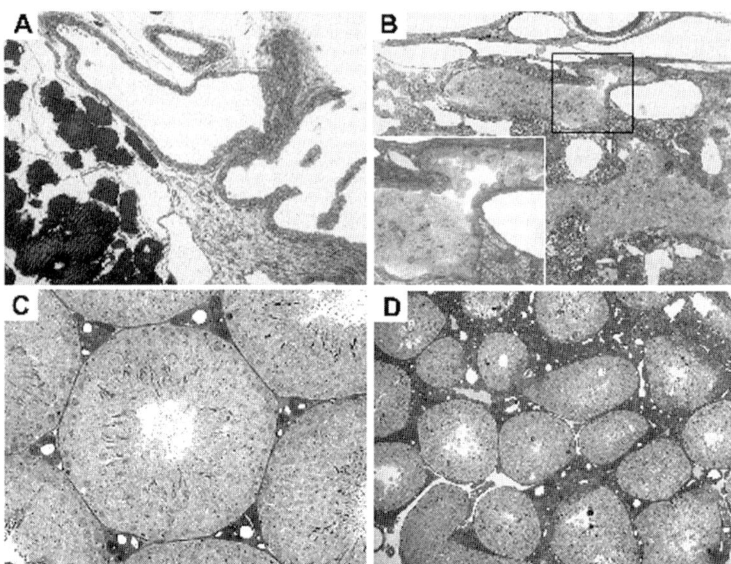

Fig. 4A–D. Light microscopic appearance of testicular sections from 12-week-old wild-type and *Dax1*-deficient male mice. **A** In the wild-type, the rete testis is a plexiform arrangement of empty spaces lined by a single cuboidal epithelial layer (×125). **B** In *Dax1*-deficient male mice, the rete testis is blocked by the proliferation of Sertoli cells (×125) accompanied by an accumulation of lipid droplets in the adjacent interstitial tissue (see insert) (×250). **C** The wild-type testis shows closely packed seminiferous tubules, a limited interstitial compartment, and complete spermatogenesis as indicated by the abundance of elongated spermatids (×250). **D** In *Dax1*-deficient male mice, the testis exhibits marked Leydig cell hyperplasia in the interstitial space (×125). (Reproduced with permission from Jeffs et al. 2001b)

knockout (KO) mice are hypogonadal and infertile, despite having normal gonadotropin production (in contrast to human AHC) and sufficient testosterone for the formation of male internal and external genitalia. Testis histology in the *Dax1* KO mice reveals progressive seminiferous tubule degeneration, loss of germ cells, impaired spermatogenesis and Leydig cell hyperplasia. In addition, tubules in the rete testis are blocked by aberrantly located Sertoli cells, creating an obstructive pathology that leads to sperm loss within the seminiferous tubules (Fig. 4). Disruption of the basement membrane in the testicular cords is accompanied by the ectopic location of poorly differentiated Leydig cells within the tubules (Jeffs et al. 2001b). Testicular biopsy findings in patients with AHC are similar to those of the animal model (Seminara et al. 1999; Ozisik et al. unpublished data).

The testicular phenotypes of knockout mice and the limited number of patients who have had testicular biopsies suggest that DAX1 plays an important role in spermatogenesis. To address the function of Dax1 more specifically, transgenic animals have been created in which the intrinsic loss of Dax1 function in either Sertoli cells or Leydig cells has been "rescued". Sertoli cell-specific expression of Dax1 was accomplished in *Dax1*-deficient male mice by using the *MIS* promoter to target expression of a *DAX1* transgene. Although testicular histology is only modestly improved in this model, fertility is restored, reflecting small improvements in sperm count and fertilizing capability (Jeffs et al. 2001a). Preliminary studies indicate that Leydig cell-specific expression of *DAX1* by the *LHR* promoter also rescues fertility in *Dax1*-deficient male mice (Meeks et al. unpublished data). Thus, the infertility associated with *Dax1*-deficiency appears to reflect combined effects on both Sertoli and Leydig cell function.

11.3 *SF1* (Steroidogenic Factor-1)

SF1 was cloned from adrenal cDNA libraries in 1992 (Lala et al. 1992). The existence of a common "steroidogenic factor" had been proposed following the identification of similar regulatory elements in the proximal promoter regions of the cytochrome P450 steroid hydroxylase gene family (Rice et al. 1991). The mouse gene encoding this protein was mapped to chromosome 2 and named *Ftzf1*, as it resembles the *Drosophila* gene, *fushi tarazu* factor 1 (FTZ-F1) (Swift and Ashworth 1995; Ueda et al. 1990). The human homologue, *FTZF1/NR5A1* contains seven exons and has been mapped to chromosome 9q33 (Taketo et al. 1995; Wong et al. 1996).

11.3.1 Structure, Expression and Function of Steroidogenic Factor-1

SF1 (*FTZF1/NR5A1*) encodes a 461 amino acid protein that is structurally similar to other members of the nuclear receptor superfamily (Fig. 5). Critical regions of SF1 include a zinc finger DBD, an A-box (or FTZF1 box), a hinge region, and an AF2 domain. The first zinc finger of SF1 contains a proximal box (P-box), which confers specificity in the recognition of DNA binding sites (Mader et al. 1989; Umesono and Evans 1989). The A-box may stabilize DNA binding (Ueda et al. 1992; Wilson et al. 1992), whereas the hinge region and the AF2 domain of SF1 are involved in transcriptional activation.

The temporal and spatial expression of *SF1* are consistent with its critical role in adrenal development, steroidogenesis, and gonadal differentiation. In the mouse, *Sf1* is first expressed in the urogenital ridge at embryonic day 9 (E9) (Hatano et al. 1994), and subsequently in the adrenal primordium (E11) and adrenal cortical cells (E13) (Morohashi et al. 1994). A similar expression pattern is seen in humans (Hanley et al. 1999; Ramayya et al. 1997). In the developing gonad, SF1 interacts with several transcription factors involved in male sex determination and testis formation (WT1, DAX1, SRY, and SOX9). In Sertoli cells, Sf1 regulates the expression of *Amh*, which leads to regression of Müllerian structures in males (Shen et al. 1994). In Leydig cells, Sf1 regulates various enzyme genes involved in steroidogenesis and testosterone biosynthesis, allowing virilization of the male fetus. In the developing ovary, *Sf1* transcript levels fall during embryogenesis in the rodent but may persist in humans (Hanley et al. 1999). Nevertheless, *Sf1* is expressed in the granulosa and theca cells of the adult ovary at the onset of folliculogenesis (Takayama et al. 1995). Finally, Sf1 also plays an important role in the development of the ventromedial hypothalamus (VMH) and pituitary gonadotropes (Ingraham et al. 1994).

SF1 regulates the transcription of a vast array of genes involved in sex determination and differentiation (*WT1, DAX1, MIS, MISR*), reproduction (*GnRHR, GSUα, LHβ, FSHR, Oxytocin, PRLR, INSL3, Inhibin α, Oct3/4*) and steroidogenesis by binding to its cognate sites in their promoters. Putative SF1 response elements have also been identified in the *FATE* (fetal and adult testis expressed transcript) promoter (Olesen et al. 2001). SF1 is believed to bind DNA as a monomer, and recognizes

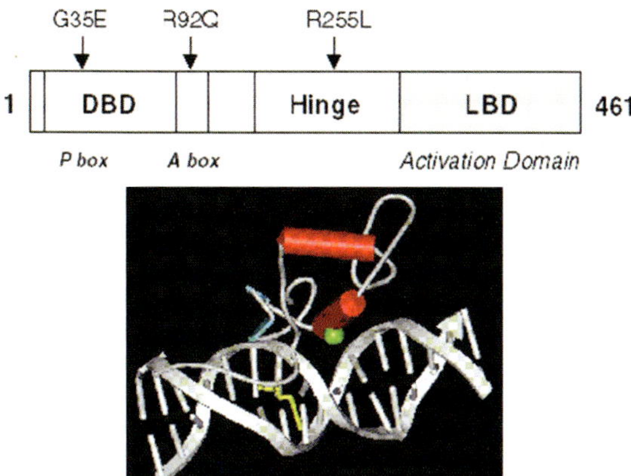

Fig. 5. A Schematic representation of SF1. DBD, LBD (which consists of an activation domain), and Hinge region are shown. The positions of the mutations G35E, R92Q, and R255L within the P-box, A-box, and Hinge region, respectively, are shown. **B** Model of SF1 binding based upon the crystal structure of nerve growth factor-induced-B (*NGFI-B*) bound to DNA as a monomer. The position of amino-acid 35 within the P-box is shown in *green* and the amino-acid 92 within the A-box is shown in *yellow*. The P-box amino acids bind to the half-site sequence (variations on AGGTCA) within the major groove of DNA, whereas the A-box is believed to bind to the 5′-flanking sequence (T/CCA) within the minor groove of DNA. (Reproduced with permission from Achermann et al. 2002)

DNA binding sites containing variations on a PyCA AGGTCA DNA sequence motif. The P-box sequence of SF1 is important in determining specificity for these response elements. The A-box (or FTZ-F1 box) may be involved in stabilizing monomeric binding, through its interaction with the PyCA of the 5'-flanking sequence. This interaction may be particularly important when DNA binding affinity is compromised following mutation of the P-box (see below) or when the target gene promoter contains a "partially conserved" half-site (Ito et al. 2000). Once bound, transactivation of target genes by SF1 involves the recruitment of coactivators such as steroid receptor coactivator-1 (SRC-1) (Ito et al. 1998), glucocorticoid receptor interacting protein (GRIP1) (Hammer et al. 1999), CREB-binding protein (CBP)/p300 (Monte et al. 1998) or proline-rich nuclear receptor coregulatory protein (PNRC) (Zhou et al. 2000). It remains unclear whether a specific ligand modulates the activation of SF1. Although oxysterols were proposed to be SF1 ligands (Lala et al. 1997), subsequent experiments showed minimal effects on transcriptional activation (Mellon and Bair 1998). It remains possible that SF1 does not require ligands for transcriptional activation. In fact, Hammer et al (Hammer et al. 1999) showed that SF1 mediated transcription can be regulated by phosphorylation of serine residue (Ser203) by the mitogen-activated protein kinase (MAPK) signaling pathway. This finding provides an additional mechanism through which SF1 may exert its actions on target genes.

11.3.2 Targeted Mutagenesis of *Sf1* (*FtzF1*)

Several groups have performed targeted deletion of *Sf1* (*FtzF1*) in mice (Luo et al. 1994; Luo et al. 1995; Sadovsky et al. 1995; Shinoda et al. 1995). Mice homozygous for the gene deletion (-/-) have complete adrenal and gonadal agenesis, male-to-female sex-reversal, and persistence of Müllerian structures in males. Adrenal failure is apparent soon after birth. A virtual absence of the hypothalamic VMH occurs and there is decreased production of gonadotropins (Ikeda et al. 1995; Shinoda et al. 1995). However, these animals are able to respond to GnRH stimulation, suggesting that Sf1 deficiency does not result in an absolute loss of gonadotropin production from the anterior pituitary (Ikeda et al. 1995). Furthermore, conditional knockout of *Sf1* in the pituitary has confirmed that the hypogonadotropic hypogonadism seen in these animals is also reversible with exogenous GnRH treatment (Zhao et al. 2001).

11.3.3 Human *SF1* (*NR5A1*) Mutations

A human *SF1* mutation was identified in a patient with primary adrenal failure, XY sex-reversal and persistent Müllerian structures (Achermann et al. 1999b). This phenotypically female patient exhibited signs of primary adrenal insufficiency during the first 2 weeks of life. Investigations prior to the induction of puberty showed a moderate gonadotropin response to GnRH stimulation and no testosterone response to exogenous hCG. Laparotomy revealed normal Müllerian structures and streak-like gonads containing poorly differentiated seminiferous tubules

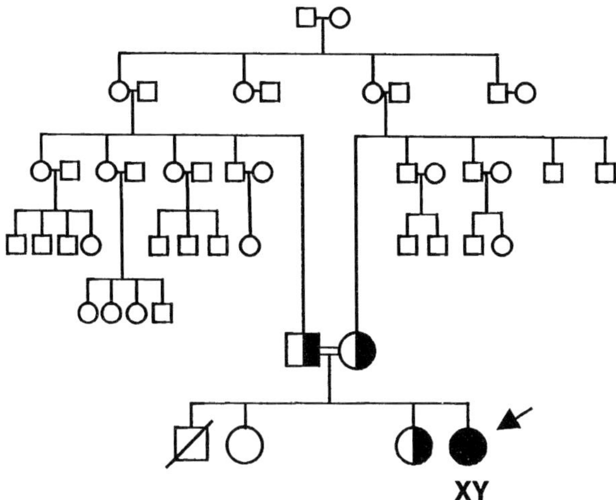

Fig. 6. Segregation of the R92Q mutation in a kindred with an SF-1 mutation. The parents are first cousins. Their first child died at 4 days of age from unknown causes. Two girls are apparently normal. The index case, shown by the *arrow*, had a hypoglycemic convulsion shortly after birth and evidence of progressive primary adrenal failure in the neonatal period. (Reproduced with permission from Achermann et al. 2002)

and connective tissue. Ethinylestradiol treatment was used to induce feminization and menstruation occurred after the introduction of cyclical progestogen, confirming the presence of a uterus. Mutation analysis revealed a de novo heterozygous G35E mutation within the P-box of the SF1 DNA-binding domain (Fig. 5). Functional studies showed that this mutation did not interfere with protein expression or nuclear localization. However, as predicted from the location of the mutation in the DNA-binding domain, the mutant SF1 failed to bind and transactivate SF1 target genes such as *Cyp11a* (*P450scc*), *Dax1*, or *LH*β (see below).

The phenotype of this patient with a heterozygous point mutation in *SF1* is less severe than the complete adrenal and gonadal agenesis seen in homozygous *Sf1* (-/-) knockout mice. Recent evidence suggests that heterozygous *Sf1* (-/+) knockout mice also exhibit impaired adrenal function, though not as severe as that seen in this patient (Bland et al. 2000). The mutant SF1 protein does not exhibit dominant negative

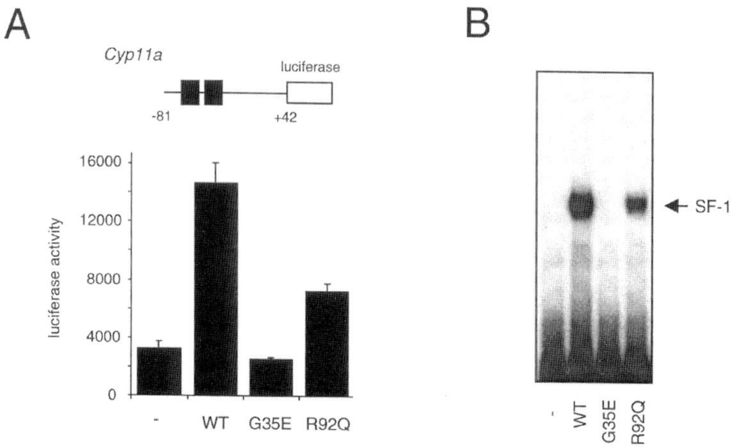

Fig. 7A, B. Functional effects of SF-1 mutations. **A** The R92Q A-box mutant shows impaired activation of a critical SF1 target gene, *Cyp11a* (P450scc), and **B** reduced binding to a probe corresponding to the SF1 binding site (TCA AGGCTA) of this promoter. However, this loss of function was not as severe as that seen with the G35E P-box mutant. (Reproduced with permission from Achermann et al. 2002)

activity (Ito et al. 2000). Therefore, it is likely that SF1 acts in a dose-dependent manner. Since SF1 regulates so many genes involved in steroidogenesis, haploinsufficiency of SF1 could have a cumulative effect on multiple steps of steroid production.

The identification of additional SF1 mutations will help to determine important structural domains of this nuclear receptor. Recently, a second de novo heterozygous SF1 mutation (R255L) was found in a XX female with adrenal insufficiency (Biason-Lauber and Schoenle 2000). This mutation affects a conserved residue in the hinge region of SF1 (Fig. 5). Although the mutation renders the molecule transcriptionally inactive, it does not appear to impair ovarian development. Whether this mutant SF1 will interfere with ovarian function at the expected time of puberty is unknown.

A homozygous *SF1* mutation has been identified in a baby born to consanguineous parents (Fig. 6) (Achermann et al., in press). This autosomal recessive mutation affects the A-box region of SF1 that modulates DNA binding by monomers (Fig. 5) (Ito et al. 2000; Wilson et al. 1993). In contrast to the P-box mutation, this A-box change (R92Q) is associated with a partial loss of function and impaired binding to its response element (Fig. 7). The surprising fact that the other family members are phenotypically normal, despite having one mutant allele reveals the exquisite sensitivity of developmental pathways to gene dosage and residual function of SF1 in humans.

11.4 Future Directions

As highlighted in this review of DAX1 and SF1, naturally-occurring mutations in humans and targeted gene disruption in mice have provided unique insights into many of the biological events involved in sexual differentiation. Despite the important advances in this field, much remains to be learned. The mechanism by which DAX1 modulates transcriptional control by SF1 and other factors is incompletely understood. The identification of additional target genes for SF1 and DAX1 will help to further unravel their physiologic roles. Many other genes are, of course, involved in the genetic pathway that leads to testis differentiation. In addition to *SRY* and *SOX9*, which genes are essential for testis determination? How are these genetic pathways regulated? Does SRY regulate SOX9 expression in a serial pathway? Or, are these genes expressed and controlled independently? Does DAX1 inhibit SRY action directly or indirectly? What are the relative functional roles of transcription factors (e.g., WT1, SF1, and SOX9) versus paracrine factors (e.g., DHH, Wnt4, MIS) in cellular differentiation and development? Presumably, extracellular signals interact with intrinsic transcription factors to regulate cell differentiation during gonadal development. Thus, a long-term goal in this field is to further characterize the genetic cascade and regulatory pathways that dictate cell fate during gonadal development.

Acknowledgements. This work received funding from the National Cooperative Program for Infertility Research and was supported by NIH Grants U54-HD-29164, PO1 HD-21921 and GCRC grant MO1-RR-00048.

References

Achermann JC, Gu WX, Kotlar TJ, Meeks JJ, Sabacan LP, Seminara SB, Habiby RL, et al (1999a) Mutational analysis of DAX1 in patients with hypogonadotropic hypogonadism or pubertal delay. J Clin Endocrinol Metab 84:4497–4500

Achermann JC, Ito M, Hindmarsh PC, Jameson JL (1999b) A mutation in the gene encoding steroidogenic factor-1 causes XY sex reversal and adrenal failure in humans. Nat Genet 22:125–126

Achermann JC, Ito M, Silverman BL, Habiby RL, Pang S, Rosler A, Jameson JL (2001) Missense mutations cluster within the carboxyl-terminal region of DAX-1 and impair transcriptional repression. J Clin Endocrinol Metab 86:3171–3175

Achermann JC, Ozisik G, Ito M, Orun UA, Harmanci K, Gurakan B, Jameson JL (2002) Gonadal determination and adrenal development are regulated by the orphan nuclear receptor, Steroidigenic Factor-1, in a dose-dependent manner. J Clin Endocrinol Metab (in press)

Albrecht KH, Eicher EM (2001) Evidence that sry is expressed in pre-Sertoli cells and Sertoli and granulosa cells have a common precursor. Dev Biol 240:92–107

Altincicek B, Tenbaum SP, Dressel U, Thormeyer D, Renkawitz R, Baniahmad A (2000) Interaction of the corepressor Alien with DAX-1 is abrogated by mutations of DAX-1 involved in adrenal hypoplasia congenita. J Biol Chem 275:7662–7667

Babu PS, Bavers DL, Beuschlein F, Shah S, Jeffs B, Jameson JL, Hammer GD (2002) Interaction Between Dax-1 and Steroidogenic Factor-1 in Vivo: Increased Adrenal Responsiveness to ACTH in the Absence of Dax-1. Endocrinology 143:665–673

Bardoni B, Zanaria E, Guioli S, Floridia G, Worley KC, Tonini G, Ferrante E, et al (1994) A dosage sensitive locus at chromosome Xp21 is involved in male to female sex reversal. Nat Genet 7:497–501

Biason-Lauber A, Schoenle EJ (2000) Apparently normal ovarian differentiation in a prepubertal girl with transcriptionally inactive steroidogenic factor 1 (NR5A1/SF-1) and adrenocortical insufficiency. Am J Hum Genet 67:1563–1568

Bland ML, Jamieson CA, Akana SF, Bornstein SR, Eisenhofer G, Dallman MF, Ingraham HA (2000) Haploinsufficiency of steroidogenic factor-1 in mice disrupts adrenal development leading to an impaired stress response. Proc Natl Acad Sci U S A 97:14488–14493

Crawford PA, Dorn C, Sadovsky Y, Milbrandt J (1998) Nuclear receptor DAX-1 recruits nuclear receptor corepressor N-CoR to steroidogenic factor 1. Mol Cell Biol 18:2949–2956

Guo W, Burris TP, McCabe ER (1995) Expression of DAX-1, the gene responsible for X-linked adrenal hypoplasia congenita and hypogonadotropic hypogonadism, in the hypothalamic-pituitary-adrenal/gonadal axis. Biochem Mol Med 56:8–13

Habiby RL, Boepple P, Nachtigall L, Sluss PM, Crowley WF, Jr., Jameson JL (1996) Adrenal hypoplasia congenita with hypogonadotropic hypogonadism: evidence that DAX-1 mutations lead to combined hypothalmic and pituitary defects in gonadotropin production. J Clin Invest 98:1055–1062

Hammer GD, Krylova I, Zhang Y, Darimont BD, Simpson K, Weigel NL, Ingraham HA (1999) Phosphorylation of the nuclear receptor SF-1 modulates cofactor recruitment: integration of hormone signaling in reproduction and stress. Mol Cell 3:521–526

Hanley NA, Ball SG, Clement-Jones M, Hagan DM, Strachan T, Lindsay S, Robson S, et al (1999) Expression of steroidogenic factor 1 and Wilms' tumour 1 during early human gonadal development and sex determination. Mech Dev 87:175–180

Hanley NA, Hagan DM, Clement-Jones M, Ball SG, Strachan T, Salas-Cortes L, McElreavey K, et al (2000) SRY, SOX9, and DAX1 expression patterns during human sex determination and gonadal development. Mech Dev 91:403–407

Hatano O, Takayama K, Imai T, Waterman MR, Takakusu A, Omura T, Morohashi K (1994) Sex-dependent expression of a transcription factor, Ad4BP, regulating steroidogenic P-450 genes in the gonads during prenatal and postnatal rat development. Development 120:2787–2797

Heery DM, Kalkhoven E, Hoare S, Parker MG (1997) A signature motif in transcriptional co-activators mediates binding to nuclear receptors. Nature 387:733–736

Ikeda Y, Luo X, Abbud R, Nilson JH, Parker KL (1995) The nuclear receptor steroidogenic factor 1 is essential for the formation of the ventromedial hypothalamic nucleus. Mol Endocrinol 9:478–486

Ikeda Y, Swain A, Weber TJ, Hentges KE, Zanaria E, Lalli E, Tamai KT, et al (1996) Steroidogenic factor 1 and Dax-1 colocalize in multiple cell lineages: potential links in endocrine development. Mol Endocrinol 10:1261–1272

Ikeda Y, Takeda Y, Shikayama T, Mukai T, Hisano S, Morohashi KI (2001) Comparative localization of Dax-1 and Ad4BP/SF-1 during development of the hypothalamic-pituitary-gonadal axis suggests their closely related and distinct functions. Dev Dyn 220:363–376

Ingraham HA, Lala DS, Ikeda Y, Luo X, Shen WH, Nachtigal MW, Abbud R, et al (1994) The nuclear receptor steroidogenic factor 1 acts at multiple levels of the reproductive axis. Genes Dev 8:2302–2312.

Ito M, Achermann JC, Jameson JL (2000) A naturally occurring steroidogenic factor-1 mutation exhibits differential binding and activation of target genes. J Biol Chem 275:31708–31714

Ito M, Yu R, Jameson JL (1997) DAX-1 inhibits SF-1-mediated transactivation via a carboxy-terminal domain that is deleted in adrenal hypoplasia congenita. Mol Cell Biol 17:1476–1483

Ito M, Yu RN, Jameson JL (1998) Steroidogenic factor-1 contains a carboxy-terminal transcriptional activation domain that interacts with steroid receptor coactivator-1. Mol Endocrinol 12:290–301

Jeffs B, Ito M, Yu RN, Martinson FA, Wang ZJ, Doglio LT, Jameson JL (2001a) Sertoli cell-specific rescue of fertility, but not testicular pathology, in Dax1 (Ahch)-deficient male mice. Endocrinology 142:2481–2488

Jeffs B, Meeks JJ, Ito M, Martinson FA, Matzuk MM, Jameson JL, Russell LD (2001b) Blockage of the rete testis and efferent ductules by ectopic Sertoli and Leydig cells causes infertility in Dax1-deficient male mice. Endocrinology 142:4486–4495

Johansson L, Bavner A, Thomsen JS, Farnegardh M, Gustafsson JA, Treuter E (2000) The orphan nuclear receptor SHP utilizes conserved LXXLL-related motifs for interactions with ligand-activated estrogen receptors. Mol Cell Biol 20:1124–1133

Kwok C, Weller PA, Guioli S, Foster JW, Mansour S, Zuffardi O, Punnett HH, et al (1995) Mutations in SOX9, the gene responsible for Campomelic dysplasia and autosomal sex reversal. Am J Hum Genet 57:1028–1036

Lala D S, Rice DA, Parker KL (1992) Steroidogenic factor I, a key regulator of steroidogenic enzyme expression, is the mouse homolog of fushi tarazufactor I. Mol Endocrinol 6:1249–1258

Lala DS, Syka PM, Lazarchik SB, Mangelsdorf DJ, Parker KL, Heyman RA (1997) Activation of the orphan nuclear receptor steroidogenic factor 1 by oxysterols. Proc Natl Acad Sci U S A 94:4895–4900

Lalli E, Bardoni B, Zazopoulos E, Wurtz JM, Strom TM, Moras D, Sassone-Corsi P (1997) A transcriptional silencing domain in DAX-1 whose mutation causes adrenal hypoplasia congenita. Mol Endocrinol 11:1950–1960

Lalli E, Ohe K, Hindelang C, Sassone-Corsi P (2000) Orphan receptor DAX-1 is a shuttling RNA binding protein associated with polyribosomes via mRNA. Mol Cell Biol 20:4910–4921

Luo X, Ikeda Y, Parker KL (1994) A cell-specific nuclear receptor is essential for adrenal and gonadal development and sexual differentiation. Cell 77:481–490

Luo X, Ikeda Y, Schlosser DA, Parker KL (1995) Steroidogenic factor 1 is the essential transcript of the mouse Ftz-F1 gene. Mol Endocrinol 9:1233–1239

MacLaughlin DT, Teixeira J, Donahoe PK (2001) Perspective: reproductive tract development–new discoveries and future directions. Endocrinology 142:2167–2172

Mader S, Kumar V, de Verneuil H, Chambon P (1989) Three amino acids of the oestrogen receptor are essential to its ability to distinguish an oestrogen from a glucocorticoid-responsive element. Nature 338:271–274

Mantovani G, Ozisik G, Achermann JC, Romoli R, Borretta G, Persani L, Spada A, et al (2002) Hypogonadotropic hypogonadism as a presenting feature of late-onset x-linked adrenal hypoplasia congenita. J Clin Endocrinol Metab 87:44–48

Mellon SH, Bair SR (1998) 25-Hydroxycholesterol is not a ligand for the orphan nuclear receptor steroidogenic factor-1 (SF-1). Endocrinology 139:3026–3029

Monte D, DeWitte F, Hum DW (1998) Regulation of the human P450scc gene by steroidogenic factor 1 is mediated by CBP/p300. J Biol Chem 273:4585–4591

Morohashi K, Iida H, Nomura M, Hatano O, Honda S, Tsukiyama T, Niwa O, et al (1994) Functional difference between Ad4BP and ELP, and their distributions in steroidogenic tissues. Mol Endocrinol 8:643–653

Muscatelli F, Strom TM, Walker AP, Zanaria E, Recan D, Meindl A, Bardoni B, et al (1994) Mutations in the DAX-1 gene give rise to both X-linked adrenal hypoplasia congenita and hypogonadotropic hypogonadism. Nature 372:672–676

Nakae J, Tajima T, Kusuda S, Kohda N, Okabe T, Shinohara N, Kato M, et al (1996) Truncation at the C-terminus of the DAX-1 protein impairs its biological actions in patients with X-linked adrenal hypoplasia congenita. J Clin Endocrinol Metab 81:3680–3685

Olesen C, Larsen NJ, Byskov AG, Harboe TL, Tommerup N (2001) Human FATE is a novel X-linked gene expressed in fetal and adult testis. Mol Cell Endocrinol 184:25–32

Phelan JK, McCabe ER (2001) Mutations in NR0B1 (DAX1) and NR5A1 (SF1) responsible for adrenal hypoplasia congenita. Hum Mutat 18:472–487

Ramayya MS, Zhou J, Kino T, Segars JH, Bondy CA, Chrousos GP (1997) Steroidogenic factor 1 messenger ribonucleic acid expression in steroidogenic and nonsteroidogenic human tissues: Northern blot and in situ hybridization studies. J Clin Endocrinol Metab 82:1799–1806

Reutens AT, Achermann JC, Ito M, Gu WX, Habiby RL, Donohoue PA, Pang S, et al (1999) Clinical and functional effects of mutations in the DAX-1 gene in patients with adrenal hypoplasia congenita. J Clin Endocrinol Metab 84:504–511

Rice DA, Mouw AR, Bogerd AM, Parker KL (1991) A shared promoter element regulates the expression of three steroidogenic enzymes. Mol Endocrinol 5:1552–1561

Sadovsky Y, Crawford PA, Woodson KG, Polish JA, Clements MA, Tourtellotte LM, Simburger K, et al (1995) Mice deficient in the orphan receptor steroidogenic factor 1 lack adrenal glands and gonads but express P450 side-chain-cleavage enzyme in the placenta and have normal embryonic serum levels of corticosteroids. Proc Natl Acad Sci U S A 92:10939–10943

Seminara SB, Achermann JC, Genel M, Jameson JL, Crowley WF, Jr. (1999) X-linked adrenal hypoplasia congenita: a mutation in DAX1 expands the phenotypic spectrum in males and females. J Clin Endocrinol Metab 84:4501–4509

Shen WH, Moore CC, Ikeda Y, Parker KL, Ingraham HA (1994) Nuclear receptor steroidogenic factor 1 regulates the mullerian inhibiting substance gene: a link to the sex determination cascade. Cell 77:651–661

Shinoda K, Lei H, Yoshii H, Nomura M, Nagano M, Shiba H, Sasaki H, et al (1995) Developmental defects of the ventromedial hypothalamic nucleus and pituitary gonadotroph in the Ftz-F1 disrupted mice. Dev Dyn 204:22–29

Swain A, Lovell-Badge R (1999) Mammalian sex determination: a molecular drama. Genes Dev 13:755–767

Swain A, Narvaez V, Burgoyne P, Camerino G, Lovell-Badge R (1998) Dax1 antagonizes Sry action in mammalian sex determination. Nature 391:761–767

Swift S, Ashworth A (1995) The mouse Ftzf1 gene required for gonadal and adrenal development maps to mouse chromosome 2. Genomics 28:609–610

Tabarin A, Achermann JC, Recan D, Bex V, Bertagna X, Christin-Maitre S, Ito M, et al (2000) A novel mutation in DAX1 causes delayed-onset adrenal insufficiency and incomplete hypogonadotropic hypogonadism. J Clin Invest 105:321–328

Takayama K, Sasano H, Fukaya T, Morohashi K, Suzuki T, Tamura M, Costa MJ, et al (1995) Immunohistochemical localization of Ad4-binding protein with correlation to steroidogenic enzyme expression in cycling human ovaries and sex cord stromal tumors. J Clin Endocrinol Metab 80:2815–2821

Taketo M, Parker KL, Howard TA, Tsukiyama T, Wong M, Niwa O, Morton CC, et al (1995) Homologs of Drosophila Fushi-Tarazu factor 1 map to mouse chromosome 2 and human chromosome 9q33. Genomics 25:565–567

Tamai KT, Monaco L, Alastalo TP, Lalli E, Parvinen M, Sassone-Corsi P (1996) Hormonal and developmental regulation of DAX-1 expression in Sertoli cells. Mol Endocrinol 10:1561–1569

Ueda H, Sonoda S, Brown JL, Scott MP, Wu C (1990) A sequence-specific DNA-binding protein that activates fushi tarazu segmentation gene expression. Genes Dev 4:624–635

Ueda H, Sun GC, Murata T, Hirose S (1992) A novel DNA-binding motif abuts the zinc finger domain of insect nuclear hormone receptor FTZ-F1 and mouse embryonal long terminal repeat-binding protein. Mol Cell Biol 12:5667–5672

Umesono K, Evans RM (1989) Determinants of target gene specificity for steroid/thyroid hormone receptors. Cell 57:1139–1146

Vidal VP, Chaboissier MC, de Rooij DG, Schedl A (2001) Sox9 induces testis development in XX transgenic mice. Nat Genet 28:216–217

Wilson TE, Fahrner TJ, Milbrandt J (1993) The orphan receptors NGFI-B and steroidogenic factor 1 establish monomer binding as a third paradigm of nuclear receptor-DNA interaction. Mol Cell Biol 13:5794–5804

Wilson TE, Paulsen RE, Padgett KA, Milbrandt J (1992) Participation of non-zinc finger residues in DNA binding by two nuclear orphan receptors. Science 256:107–110

Wong M, Ramayya MS, Chrousos GP, Driggers PH, Parker KL (1996) Cloning and sequence analysis of the human gene encoding steroidogenic factor 1. J Mol Endocrinol 17:139–47.

Yu RN, Ito M, Saunders TL, Camper SA, Jameson JL (1998) Role of Ahch in gonadal development and gametogenesis. Nat Genet 20:353–357

Zhang H, Thomsen JS, Johansson L, Gustafsson JA, Treuter E (2000) DAX-1 functions as an LXXLL-containing corepressor for activated estrogen receptors. J Biol Chem 275:39855–39859

Zhang YH, Guo W, Wagner RL, Huang BL, McCabe L, Vilain E, Burris TP, et al (1998) DAX1 mutations map to putative structural domains in a deduced three-dimensional model. Am J Hum Genet 62:855–864

Zhao L, Bakke M, Krimkevich Y, Cushman LJ, Parlow AF, Camper SA, Parker KL (2001) Steroidogenic factor 1 (SF1) is essential for pituitary gonadotrope function. Development 128:147–154

Zhou D, Quach KM, Yang C, Lee SY, Pohajdak B, Chen S (2000) PNRC: a proline-rich nuclear receptor coregulatory protein that modulates transcriptional activation of multiple nuclear receptors including orphan receptors SF1 (steroidogenic factor 1) and ERRalpha1 (estrogen related receptor alpha-1). Mol Endocrinol 14:986–998

Ernst Schering Research Foundation Workshop

Editors: Günter Stock
             Monika Lessl

Vol. 1 *(1991)*: Bioscience ⇆ Society – Workshop Report
Editors: D. J. Roy, B. E. Wynne, R. W. Old

Vol. 2 (1991): Round Table Discussion on Bioscience ⇆ Society
Editor: J. J. Cherfas

Vol. 3 (1991): Excitatory Amino Acids and Second Messenger Systems
Editors: V. I. Teichberg, L. Turski

Vol. 4 (1992): Spermatogenesis – Fertilization – Contraception
Editors: E. Nieschlag, U.-F. Habenicht

Vol. 5 (1992): Sex Steroids and the Cardiovascular System
Editors: P. Ramwell, G. Rubanyi, E. Schillinger

Vol. 6 (1993): Transgenic Animals as Model Systems for Human Diseases
Editors: E. F. Wagner, F. Theuring

Vol. 7 (1993): Basic Mechanisms Controlling Term and Preterm Birth
Editors: K. Chwalisz, R. E. Garfield

Vol. 8 (1994): Health Care 2010
Editors: C. Bezold, K. Knabner

Vol. 9 (1994): Sex Steroids and Bone
Editors: R. Ziegler, J. Pfeilschifter, M. Bräutigam

Vol. 10 (1994): Nongenotoxic Carcinogenesis
Editors: A. Cockburn, L. Smith

Vol. 11 (1994): Cell Culture in Pharmaceutical Research
Editors: N. E. Fusenig, H. Graf

Vol. 12 (1994): Interactions Between Adjuvants, Agrochemical
and Target Organisms
Editors: P. J. Holloway, R. T. Rees, D. Stock

Vol. 13 (1994): Assessment of the Use of Single Cytochrome
P450 Enzymes in Drug Research
Editors: M. R. Waterman, M. Hildebrand

Vol. 14 (1995): Apoptosis in Hormone-Dependent Cancers
Editors: M. Tenniswood, H. Michna

Vol. 15 (1995): Computer Aided Drug Design in Industrial Research
Editors: E. C. Herrmann, R. Franke

Vol. 16 (1995): Organ-Selective Actions of Steroid Hormones
Editors: D. T. Baird, G. Schütz, R. Krattenmacher

Vol. 17 (1996): Alzheimer's Disease
Editors: J.D. Turner, K. Beyreuther, F. Theuring

Vol. 18 (1997): The Endometrium as a Target for Contraception
Editors: H.M. Beier, M.J.K. Harper, K. Chwalisz

Vol. 19 (1997): EGF Receptor in Tumor Growth and Progression
Editors: R. B. Lichtner, R. N. Harkins

Vol. 20 (1997): Cellular Therapy
Editors: H. Wekerle, H. Graf, J.D. Turner

Vol. 21 (1997): Nitric Oxide, Cytochromes P 450,
and Sexual Steroid Hormones
Editors: J.R. Lancaster, J.F. Parkinson

Vol. 22 (1997): Impact of Molecular Biology
and New Technical Developments in Diagnostic Imaging
Editors: W. Semmler, M. Schwaiger

Vol. 23 (1998): Excitatory Amino Acids
Editors: P.H. Seeburg, I. Bresink, L. Turski

Vol. 24 (1998): Molecular Basis of Sex Hormone Receptor Function
Editors: H. Gronemeyer, U. Fuhrmann, K. Parczyk

Vol. 25 (1998): Novel Approaches to Treatment of Osteoporosis
Editors: R.G.G. Russell, T.M. Skerry, U. Kollenkirchen

Vol. 26 (1998): Recent Trends in Molecular Recognition
Editors: F. Diederich, H. Künzer

Vol. 27 (1998): Gene Therapy
Editors: R.E. Sobol, K.J. Scanlon, E. Nestaas, T. Strohmeyer

Vol. 28 (1999): Therapeutic Angiogenesis
Editors: J.A. Dormandy, W.P. Dole, G.M. Rubanyi

Vol. 29 (2000): Of Fish, Fly, Worm and Man
Editors: C. Nüsslein-Volhard, J. Krätzschmar

Vol. 30 (2000): Therapeutic Vaccination Therapy
Editors: P. Walden, W. Sterry, H. Hennekes

Vol. 31 (2000): Advances in Eicosanoid Research
Editors: C.N. Serhan, H.D. Perez

Vol. 32 (2000): The Role of Natural Products in Drug Discovery
Editors: J. Mulzer, R. Bohlmann

Supplement 1 (1994): Molecular and Cellular Endocrinology of the Testis
Editors: G. Verhoeven, U.-F. Habenicht

Supplement 2 (1997): Signal Transduction in Testicular Cells
Editors: V. Hansson, F. O. Levy, K. Taskén

Supplement 3 (1998): Testicular Function:
From Gene Expression to Genetic Manipulation
Editors: M. Stefanini, C. Boitani, M. Galdieri, R. Geremia, F. Palombi

Supplement 4 (2000): Hormone Replacement Therapy
and Osteoporosis
Editors: J. Kato, H. Minaguchi, Y. Nishino

Supplement 5 (1999): Interferon:
The Dawn of Recombinant Protein Drugs
Editors: J. Lindenmann, W.D. Schleuning

Supplement 6 (2000): Testis, Epididymis and Technologies
in the Year 2000
Editors: B. Jégou, C. Pineau, J. Saez

Supplement 7 (2001): New Concepts in Pathology and Treatment
of Autoimmune Disorders
Editors: P. Pozzilli, C. Pozzilli, J.-F. Kapp

Supplement 8 (2001): New Pharmacological Approaches
to Reproductive Health and Healthy Ageing
Editors: W.-K. Raff, M. F. Fathalla, F. Saad